Generis
PUBLISHING

The Dilemma and Outlet of Medicine

Li Xiaoguang

Title: The Dilemma and Outlet of Medicine

ISBN: 979-8-88676-189-4

Author: Li Xiaoguang

Cover image: www.pixabay.com

Publisher: Generis Publishing
Online orders: www.generis-publishing.com
Contact email: info@generis-publishing.com

Abstract

This book is a collection of the author'papers. It collects four papers published by the author since September 2020. The titles of these four papers are The Dilemma and Outlet of Modern Medicine and Opening up a New Field of Modern Medical Research.

At present, modern medicine is facing the dilemma that a large number of diseases are difficult to cure and medical treatment is expensive. These four papers put forward solutions and outlets according to the author's research and experience.

Contents

Paper 1: The Dilemma and Outlet of Modern Medicine and a Case of Asthma Successfully Cured with Herbs 7

Paper 2: Opening up a New Field of Modern Medical Research 2 29

Paper 3: Opening up a New Field of Modern Medical Research 1 41

Paper 4: Opening up a New Field of Modern Medical Research 3 75

Paper 1: The Dilemma and Outlet of Modern Medicine and a Case of Asthma Successfully Cured with Herbs

This article was published in International Journal of Clinical Studies and Medical Case Reports on May 27th, 2022. DOI: 10.46998/IJCMCR.2022.20.000478. Citation: LI Xiaoguang*. The Dilemma and Outlet of Modern Medicine and a Case of Asthma Successfully Cured with Herbs. IJCMCR. 2022; 20 (1): 002

Abstract

At present, modern medicine is faced with the dilemma that a large number of diseases can't be cured and the treatment cost is expensive. Based on the author's research and experience, this paper discusses the solutions and outlets. Asthma is a serious and potentially fatal disease, this paper introduces a case that the author successfully cured it with herbs.

Keywords

Modern medicine, traditional Chinese medicine, herbs, meridians, acupoints, asthma, ephedra.

Humans will get sick, and the types of diseases are very numerous and complex. The history of human research and treatment of diseases is also very long. Different medicine has been formed in different areas, and they have different understandings of human body and take different treatment methods for diseases. Among them, the medicine in Europe has developed by leaps and bounds with the help of the progress of modern science and technology in recent centuries, and has been spread to all countries in the world, becoming the world medicine and mainstream medicine, now it is also called modern medicine. While the medicine in other regions still exists in some areas, and is called traditional medicine, complementary medicine or alternative medicine.

Modern medicine's research and understanding of the human body has been very thorough and meticulous, reaching the molecular level, but the diseases that modern medicine can really cure are relatively few, and most of human diseases are still difficult to cure by modern medicine. This is a dilemma that modern medicine is currently facing. And at the same time, modern medicine is also facing another dilemma, that is, increasingly expensive medical expenses, which are a heavy burden for individuals, society and the government. So what is the solution and way out?

Since childhood, the author was weak and prone to illness. At the age of twelve, he began to suffer from rheumatism, and every time he got sick, he had to be treated for one or two months before he could recover. Later, he suffered from unexplained fever, gastritis, gastroptosis and asthma, which are difficult to cure with modern medicine. So the author pinned his hopes on traditional Chinese medicine, but after looking for many doctors of traditional Chinese medicine to treat him, the author was disappointed again, because it didn't have a good effect either. Fortunately, the author is good at science and likes research, so he has embarked on the road of studying traditional Chinese medicine since he was eighteen, because the author intuitively felts that traditional Chinese medicine is a potential medicine. Traditional Chinese medicine has many unique understandings of human body that modern medicine does not have, and it also has unique treatments for diseases. The later results proved that the author's judgment is correct, because these diseases of the author have been cured one after another. Asthma is cured with herbs, while other diseases are cured by massaging meridians and acupoints.

There are some herbs for treating asthma and cough in traditional Chinese medicine, but because traditional Chinese medicine doesn't completely distinguish asthma and cough in theory, it doesn't distinguish herbs for treating asthma and cough, instead, they are collectively referred to as medicines for treating asthma and cough. While In fact, asthma and cough are two diseases with completely opposite mechanisms, and anti-asthma drugs and anti-cough drugs are also two drugs with completely opposite effects, but traditional Chinese medicine often uses them at the same time clinically. Because the effects cancel each other out, the therapeutic effect is not good. And the author found out the herb which has the effect of treating asthma through his own experiments, this herb is ephedra. The author boiled 10 grams of ephedra with water, and drank it after cooling. Twice a day, he cured his asthma in only two days, and it never recurred for more than 30 years.

Asthma is a very serious and potentially fatal disease. It is said that there are 300 million patients all over the world. Author hope his experience can bring them good news.

Meridians and acupoints are the unique understanding of the human body in traditional Chinese medicine, and acupuncture and massage are also the unique treatment methods in traditional Chinese medicine. Traditional Chinese medicine believes that the human body has some vertical lines, and there are some points on these lines, which can be stimulated by acupuncture and massage to treat diseases. They are called Jingluo and Shuxue in Chinese and meridians and acupoints in English. However, traditional Chinese medicine is not very clear about the function on human body and therapeutic principle of these lines and points, and the discussion is vague, so the therapeutic effect of using them is generally not very good. Through more than 30 years' personal experiments, the author has made some new discoveries about the functions on the human body and therapeutic principles of these lines and points, so he can use them to cure some of his own diseases.

The author's new discoveries about the functions and therapeutic principles of meridians and acupoints have been published through the paper "Opening up a New Field of Modern Medical Research" [1,2] and the book "The Previously Unknown Secrets of the Human Body" [3].

From the above, we can see the importance of traditional Chinese medicine, which is the way to solve the dilemma faced by modern medicine at present. In 2015, Ms. Tu Youyou won the Nobel Prize in Medicine for discovering that artemisinin can treat malaria, she was also inspired by the experience of traditional Chinese medicine.

Traditional Chinese medicine has a history of more than 2000 years. It not only has some wrong and outdated understanding of the human body, but also has some valuable discoveries that can make up for the deficiency of modern medicine. Meridians and acupoints are very important parts, and they are also the main research objects of the author. According to the author's research and experience, as long as we make clear the functions on human body and treatment principles of meridians and acupoints, a large number of diseases of human body can be treated with them, and the method is simple and the cost is low.

The following is the distribution map of main meridians and acupoints of human body after the author's correction.

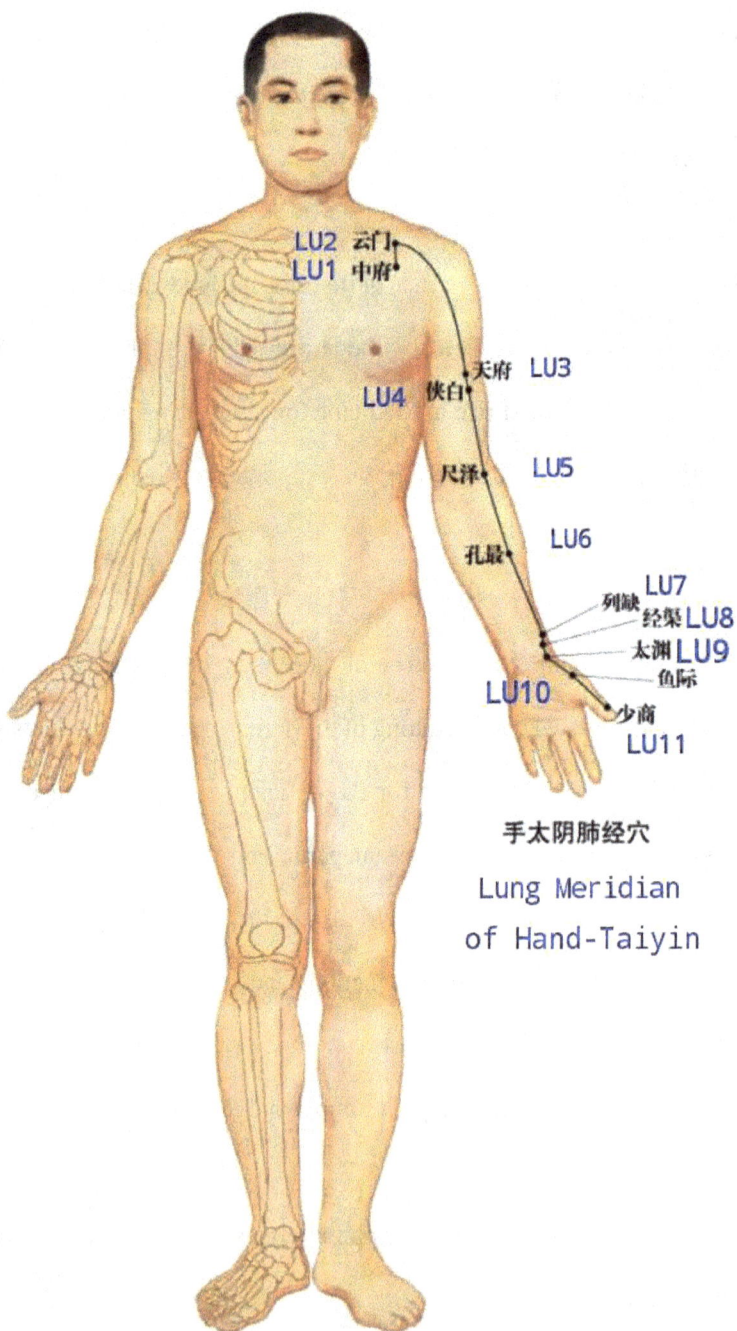

LU2 云门
LU1 中府

天府 LU3
侠白
LU4

尺泽 LU5

孔最 LU6

LU7
列缺
经渠 LU8
太渊 LU9
鱼际
LU10
少商
LU11

手太阴肺经穴

Lung Meridian
of Hand-Taiyin

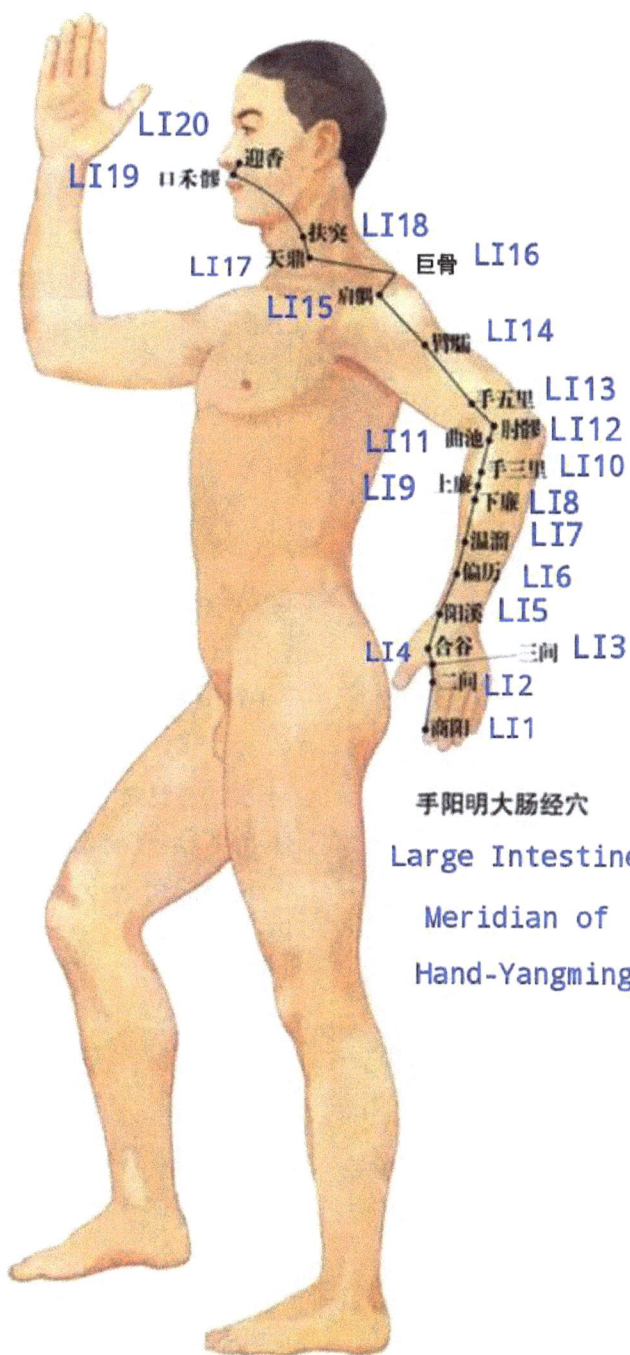

LI20 迎香
LI19 口禾髎
LI18 扶突
巨骨 LI16
LI17 天鼎
LI15 肩髃
臂臑 LI14
手五里 LI13
曲池 肘髎 LI12
LI11 手三里 LI10
LI9 上廉
下廉 LI8
温溜 LI7
偏历 LI6
阳溪 LI5
LI4 合谷 三间 LI3
二间 LI2
商阳 LI1

手阳明大肠经穴

Large Intestine
Meridian of
Hand-Yangming

13

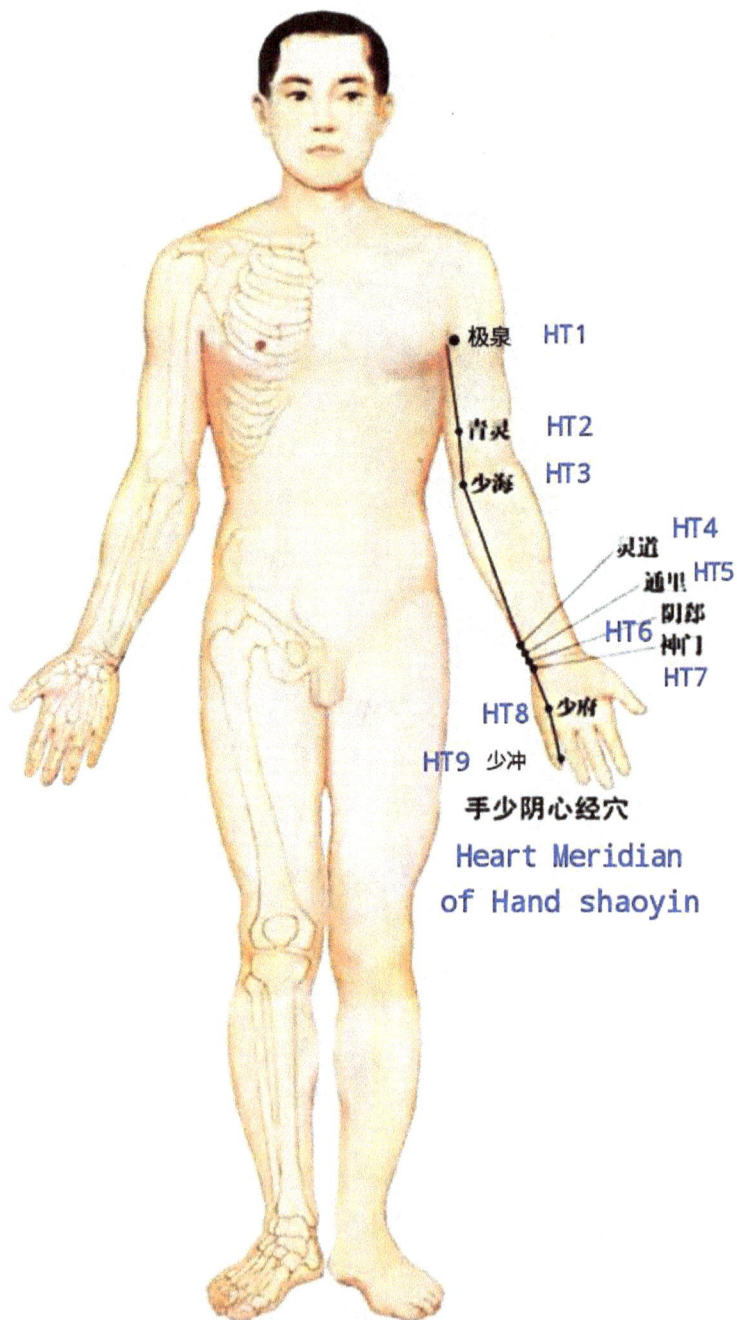

极泉　HT1

青灵　HT2
少海　HT3

灵道　HT4
通里　HT5
阴郄　HT6
神门　HT7

HT8　少府
HT9　少冲

手少阴心经穴
Heart Meridian
of Hand shaoyin

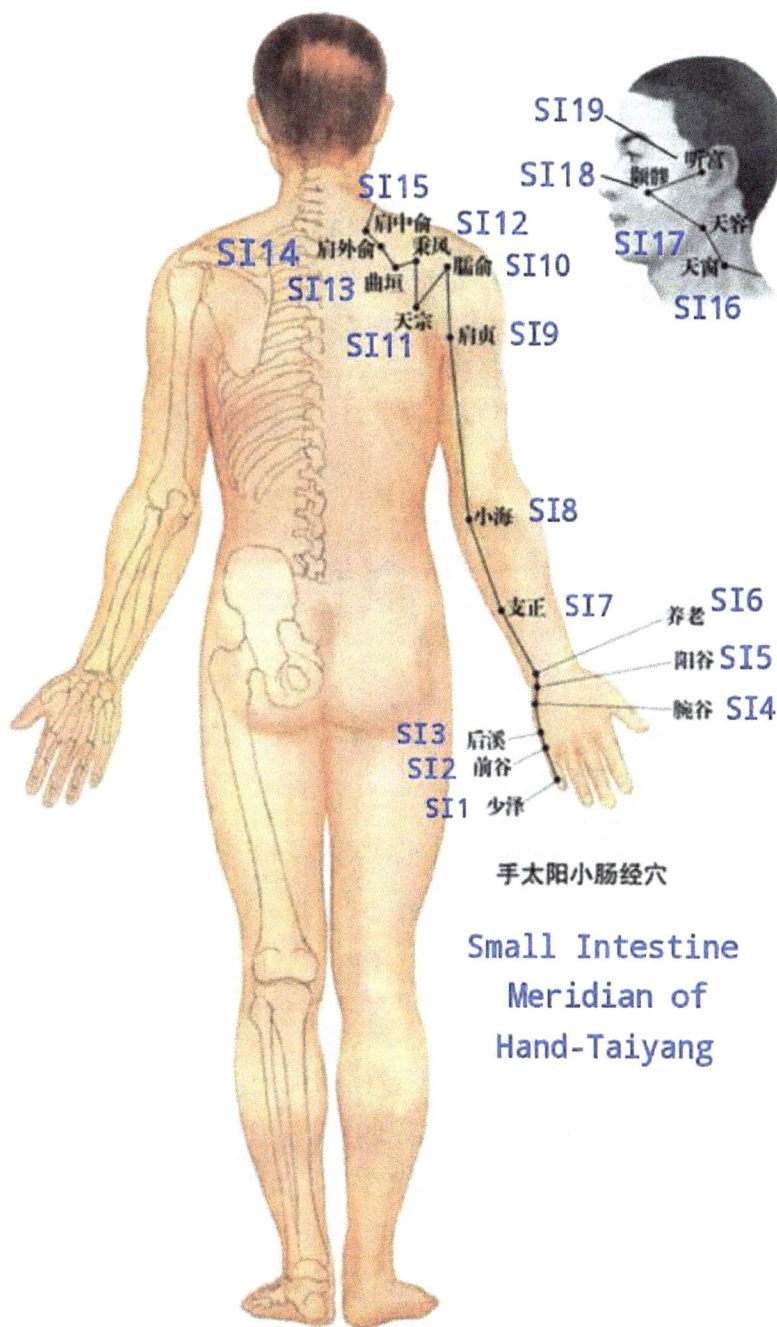

SI19 听宫
SI18 颧髎
SI17 天容
天窗
SI16

SI15 肩中俞
SI12
肩外俞 秉风
SI14 曲垣 臑俞 SI10
SI13 天宗
SI11 肩贞 SI9

小海 SI8

支正 SI7
养老 SI6
阳谷 SI5
腕谷 SI4

SI3 后溪
SI2 前谷
SI1 少泽

手太阳小肠经穴

Small Intestine
Meridian of
Hand-Taiyang

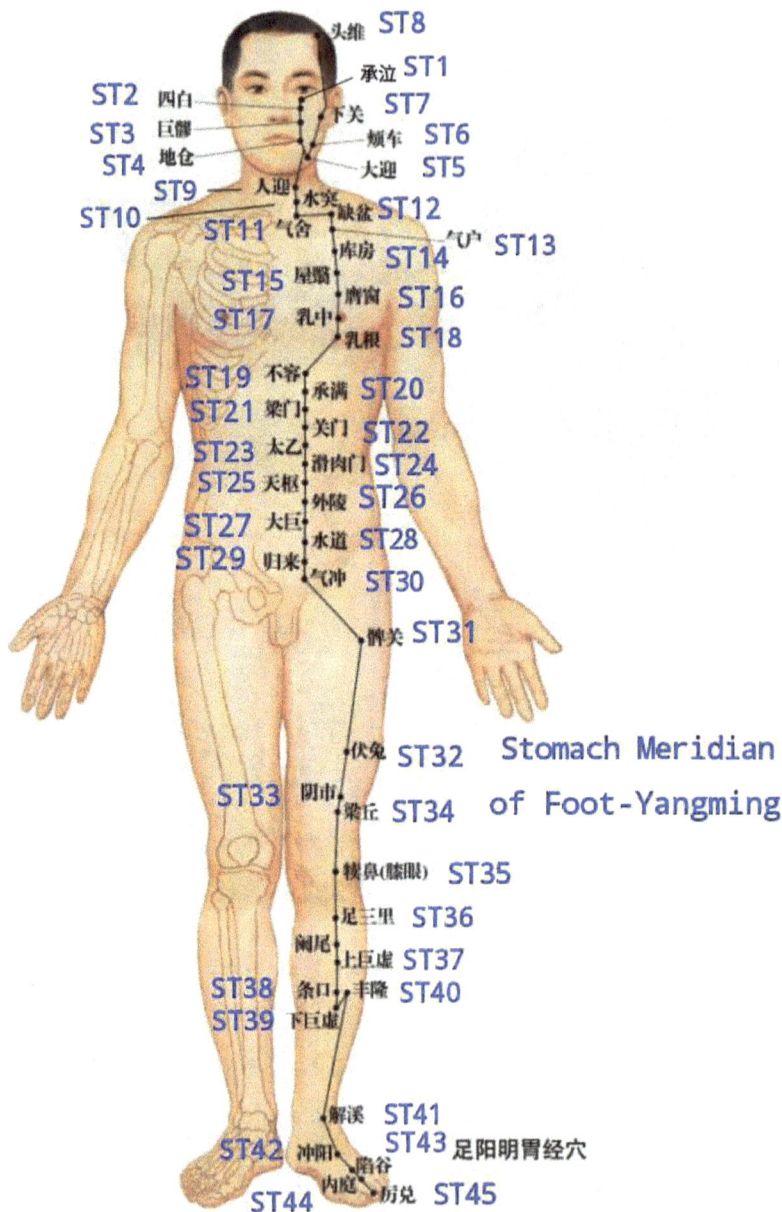

ST8 头维
ST1 承泣
ST2 四白
ST7 下关
ST3 巨髎
ST6 颊车
ST4 地仓
ST5 大迎
ST9 人迎
ST10 水突
ST12 缺盆
ST11 气舍
ST13 气户
ST14 库房
ST15 屋翳
ST16 膺窗
ST17 乳中
ST18 乳根
ST19 不容
ST20 承满
ST21 梁门
ST22 关门
ST23 太乙
ST24 滑肉门
ST25 天枢
ST26 外陵
ST27 大巨
ST28 水道
ST29 归来
ST30 气冲
ST31 髀关
ST32 伏兔
ST33 阴市
ST34 梁丘
ST35 犊鼻(膝眼)
ST36 足三里
ST37 上巨虚
阑尾
ST38 条口
ST40 丰隆
ST39 下巨虚
ST41 解溪
ST42 冲阳
ST43 陷谷
足阳明胃经穴
ST44 内庭
ST45 厉兑

Stomach Meridian
of Foot-Yangming

16

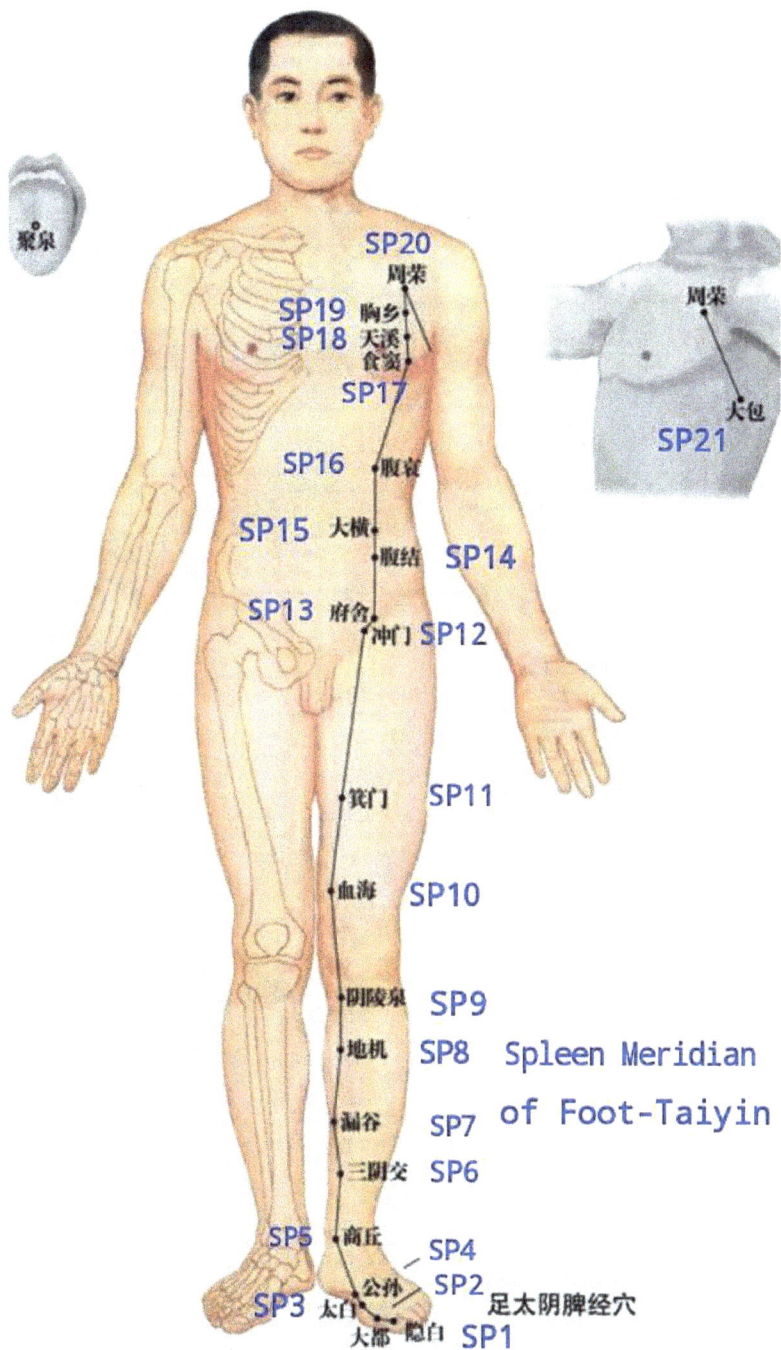

聚泉

SP20 周荣
SP19 胸乡
SP18 天溪
食窦
SP17
SP16 腹哀
SP15 大横
腹结 SP14
SP13 府舍
冲门 SP12

周荣
天包
SP21

箕门 SP11

血海 SP10

阴陵泉 SP9
地机 SP8 Spleen Meridian
漏谷 SP7 of Foot-Taiyin
三阴交 SP6
SP5 商丘 SP4
公孙 SP2
SP3 太白 足太阴脾经穴
大都 隐白 SP1

Liver Meridian
of Foot-Jueyin

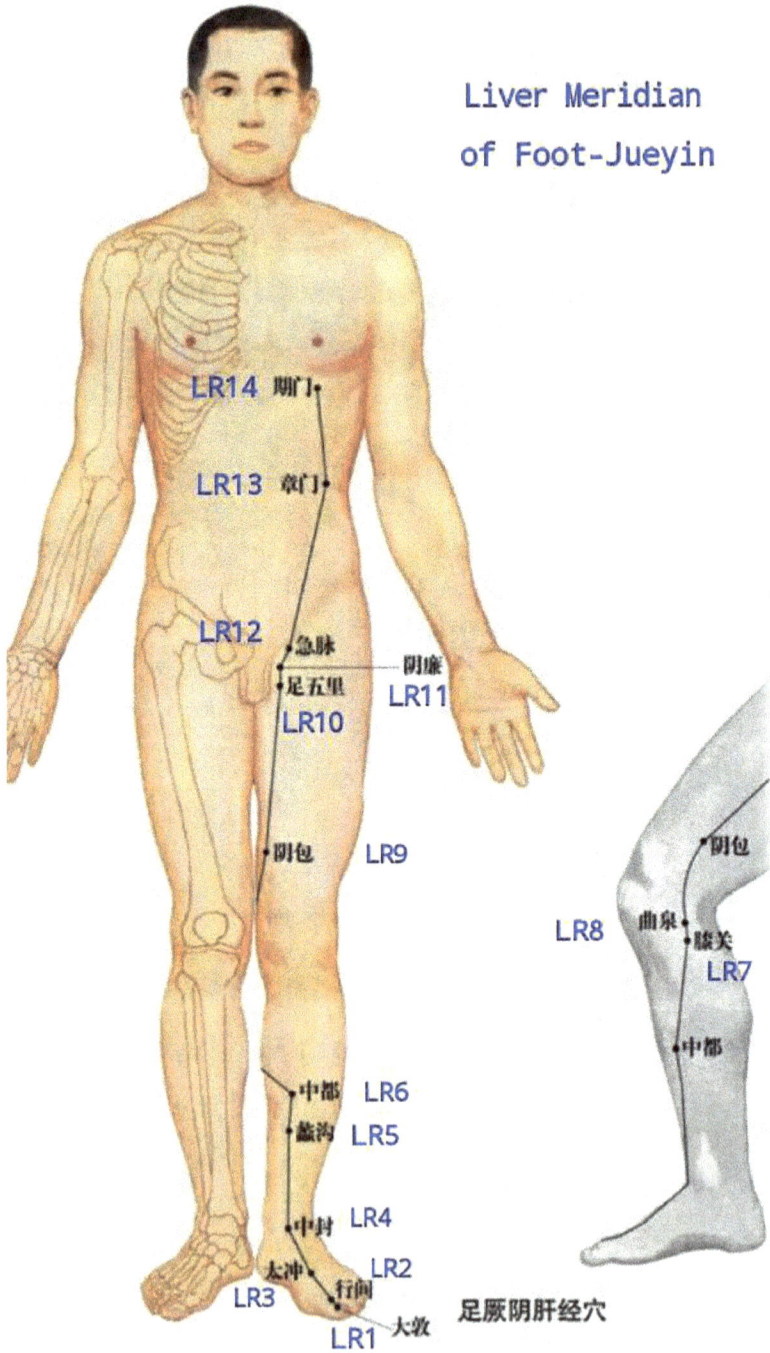

LR14 期门

LR13 章门

LR12

急脉
阴廉
足五里 LR11
LR10

阴包 LR9

阴包
曲泉
膝关
LR8 LR7

中都

中都 LR6
蠡沟 LR5

中封 LR4
太冲 LR2
行间
LR3
LR1 大敦

足厥阴肝经穴

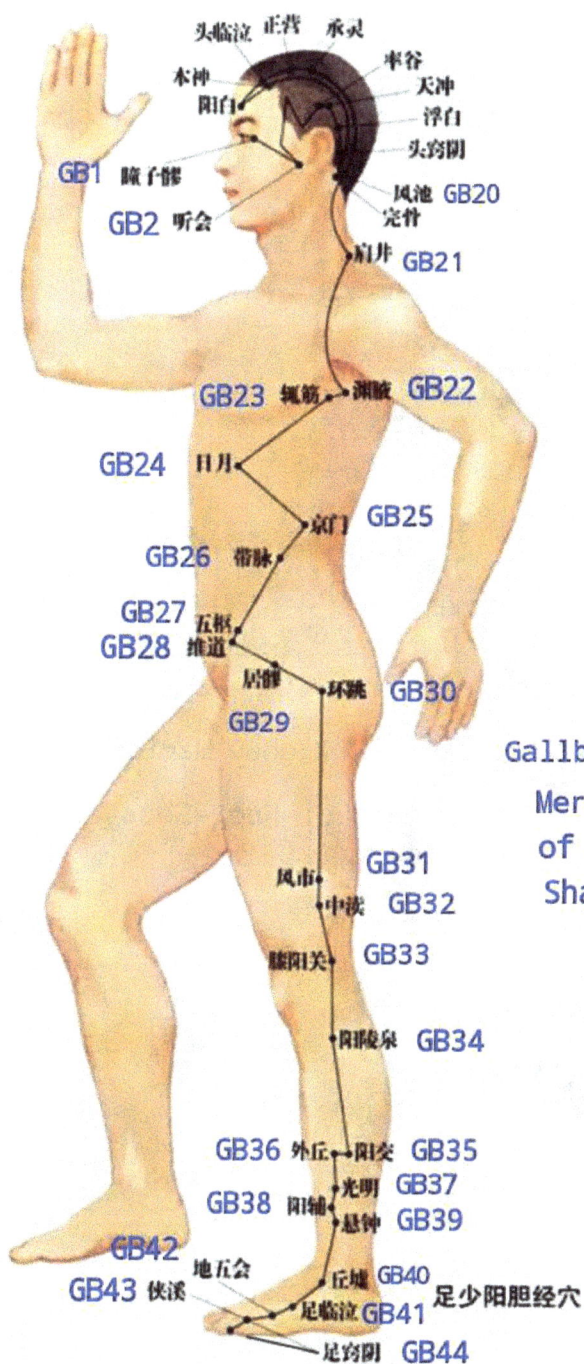

头临泣 正营 承灵
本神 率谷
阳白 天冲
浮白
头窍阴
GB1 瞳子髎 风池 GB20
完骨
GB2 听会
肩井 GB21
GB23 辄筋 渊腋 GB22
GB24 日月
京门 GB25
GB26 带脉
GB27 五枢
GB28 维道
居髎 环跳 GB30
GB29
Gallbladder
Meridian
of Foot-
Shaoyang
风市 GB31
中渎 GB32
膝阳关 GB33
阳陵泉 GB34
GB36 外丘 阳交 GB35
光明 GB37
GB38 阳辅 悬钟 GB39
GB42
地五会 丘墟 GB40
GB43 侠溪 足少阳胆经穴
足临泣 GB41
足窍阴 GB44

19

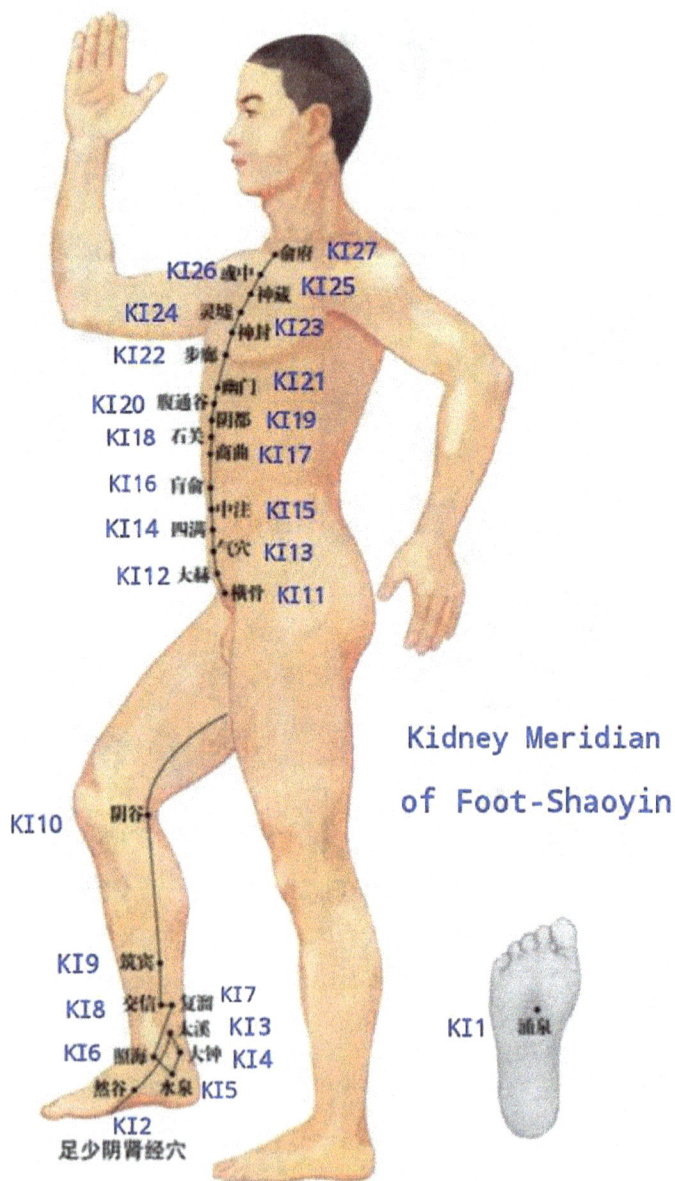

KI27 俞府
KI26 彧中
KI25 神藏
KI24 灵墟
KI23 神封
KI22 步廊
KI21 幽门
KI20 腹通谷
KI19 阴都
KI18 石关
KI17 商曲
KI16 肓俞
KI15 中注
KI14 四满
KI13 气穴
KI12 大赫
KI11 横骨

Kidney Meridian
of Foot-Shaoyin

KI10 阴谷

KI9 筑宾
KI8 交信
KI7 复溜
KI6 照海
KI3 太溪
KI4 大钟
KI5 水泉
KI2 然谷
足少阴肾经穴

KI1 涌泉

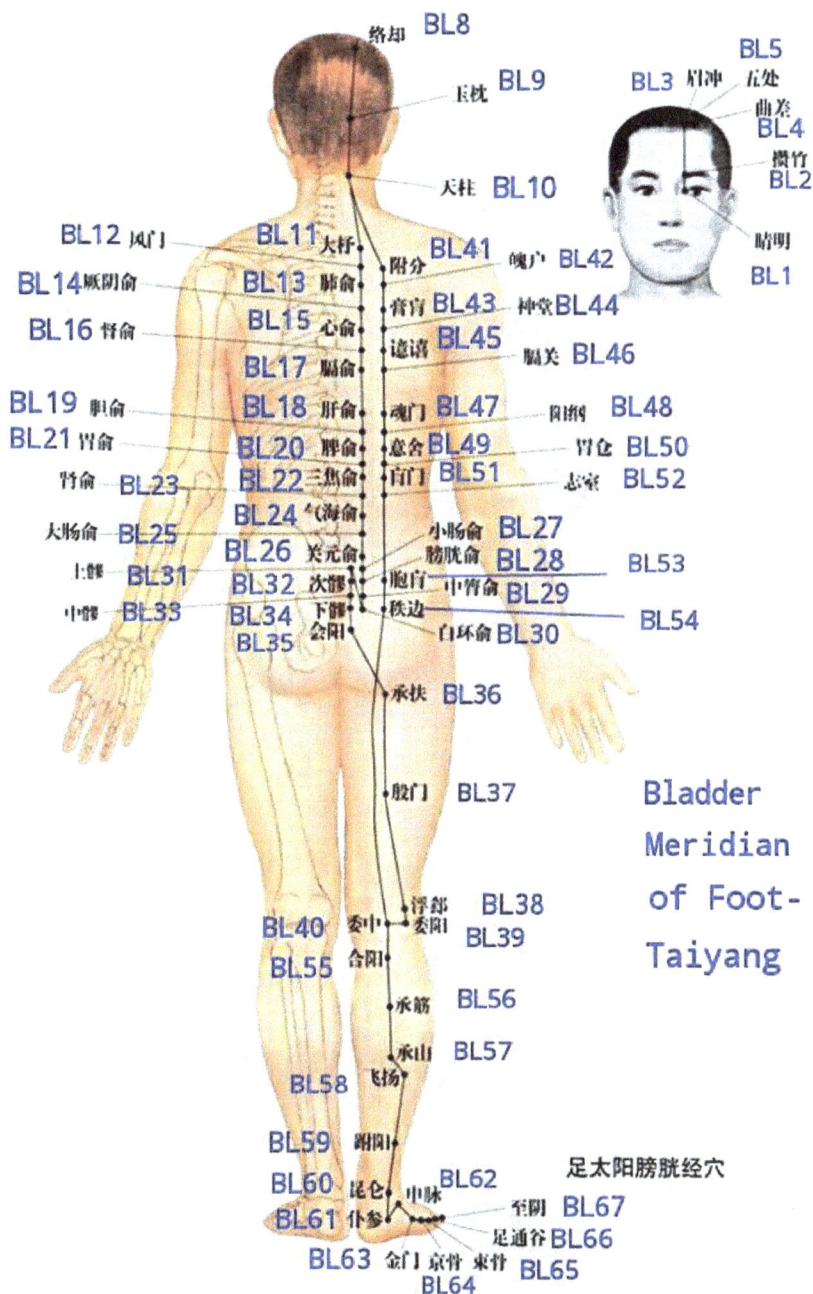

BL8 络却
BL9 玉枕
BL3 眉冲 BL5 五处
BL4 曲差
BL2 攒竹
BL1 睛明
BL10 天柱
BL11 大杼
BL12 风门
BL41 附分
BL42 魄户
BL14 厥阴俞
BL13 肺俞
BL43 膏肓 BL44 神堂
BL16 肾俞
BL15 心俞
BL45 谚谱 BL46 膈关
BL17 膈俞
BL19 胆俞
BL18 肝俞
BL47 魂门 BL48 阳纲
BL21 胃俞
BL20 脾俞
BL49 意舍 BL50 胃仓
BL22 三焦俞
BL23 肾俞
BL51 肓门 BL52 志室
BL24 气海俞
BL25 大肠俞
BL27 小肠俞
BL28 膀胱俞
BL53 胞肓
BL26 关元俞
BL31 上髎
BL32 次髎
BL29 中膂俞
BL54 秩边
BL33 中髎
BL34 下髎
BL30 白环俞 胞肓
BL35 会阳
BL36 承扶
BL37 殷门
BL38 浮郄
BL40 委中
BL39 委阳
BL55 合阳
BL56 承筋
BL57 承山
BL58 飞扬
BL59 跗阳
BL60 昆仑
BL62 申脉
BL61 仆参
BL67 至阴
BL66 足通谷
BL63 金门 京骨 束骨
BL64 BL65

Bladder Meridian of Foot- Taiyang

足太阳膀胱经穴

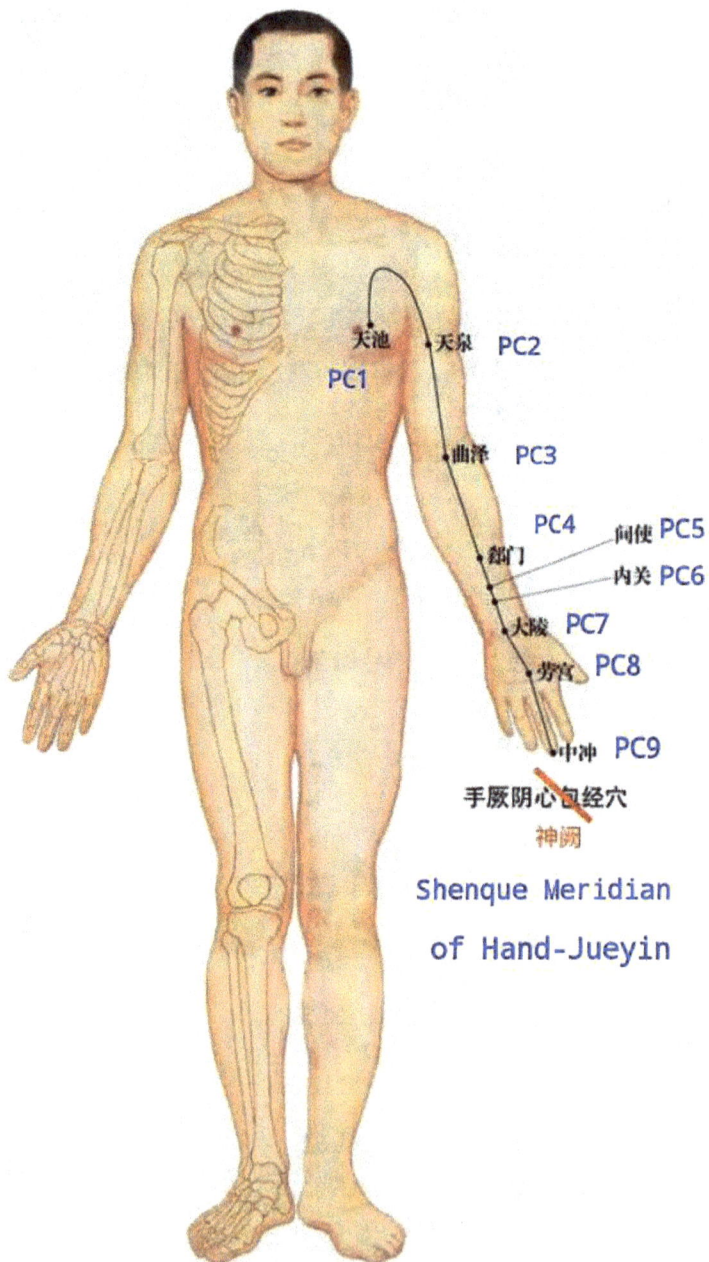

天池 天泉 PC2
PC1
曲泽 PC3
PC4 间使 PC5
郄门 内关 PC6
大陵 PC7
劳宫 PC8
中冲 PC9
手厥阴心包经穴
神阙

Shenque Meridian
of Hand-Jueyin

22

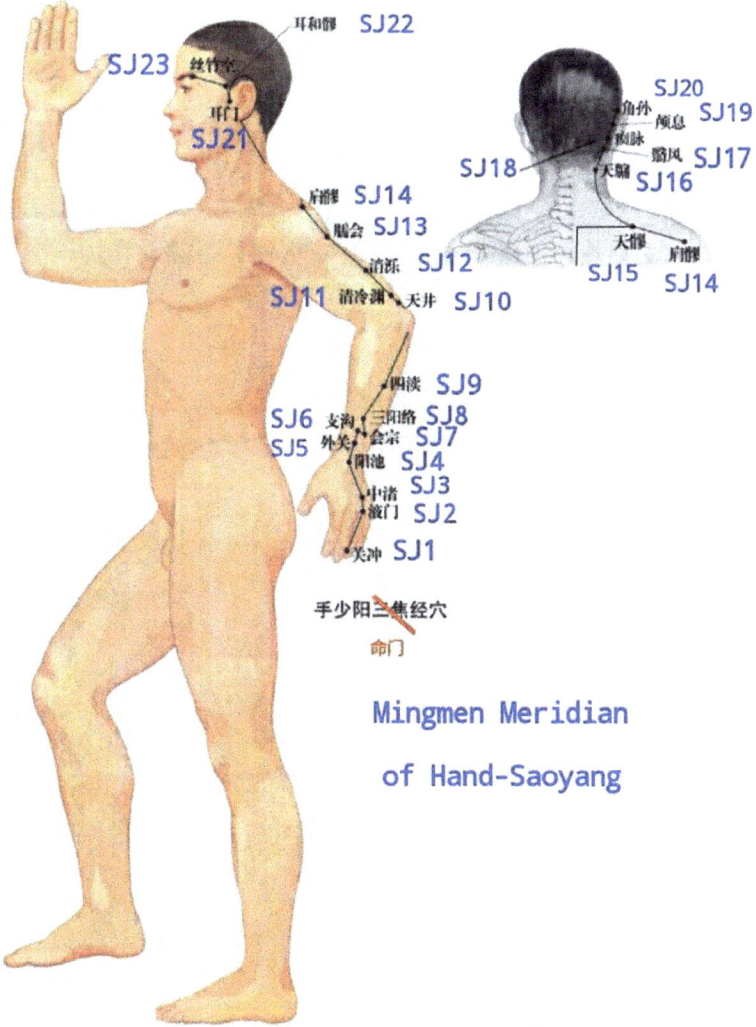

耳和髎 SJ22

SJ23

丝竹空

SJ20

角孙

颅息 SJ19

耳门

瘈脉

翳风 SJ17

SJ21

SJ18

天牖

SJ16

肩髎 SJ14

天髎

肩髎

臑会 SJ13

SJ15

SJ14

消泺 SJ12

SJ11 清冷渊 天井 SJ10

四渎 SJ9

SJ6 支沟 三阳络 SJ8

SJ5 外关 会宗 SJ7

阳池 SJ4

中渚 SJ3

液门 SJ2

关冲 SJ1

手少阳三焦经穴

命门

Mingmen Meridian

of Hand-Saoyang

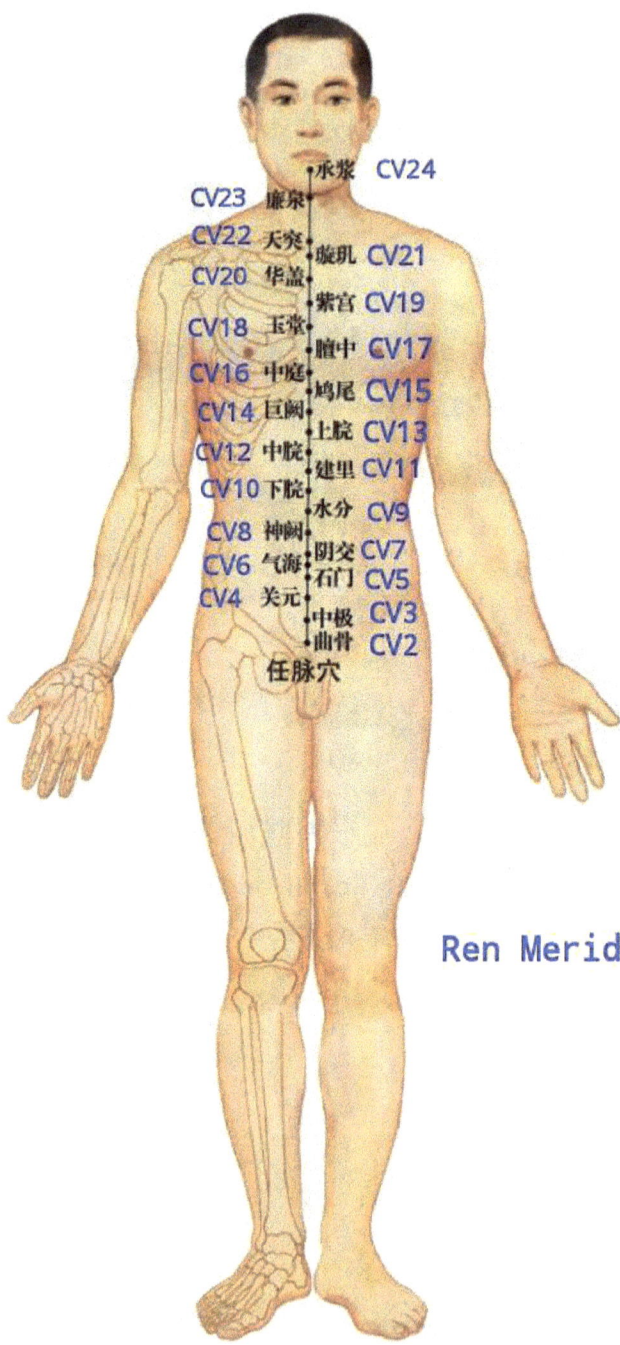

CV24 承浆
CV23 廉泉
CV22 天突
CV21 璇玑
CV20 华盖
CV19 紫宫
CV18 玉堂
CV17 膻中
CV16 中庭
CV15 鸠尾
CV14 巨阙
CV13 上脘
CV12 中脘
CV11 建里
CV10 下脘
CV9 水分
CV8 神阙
CV7 阴交
CV6 气海
CV5 石门
CV4 关元
CV3 中极
CV2 曲骨

任脉穴

Ren Meridian

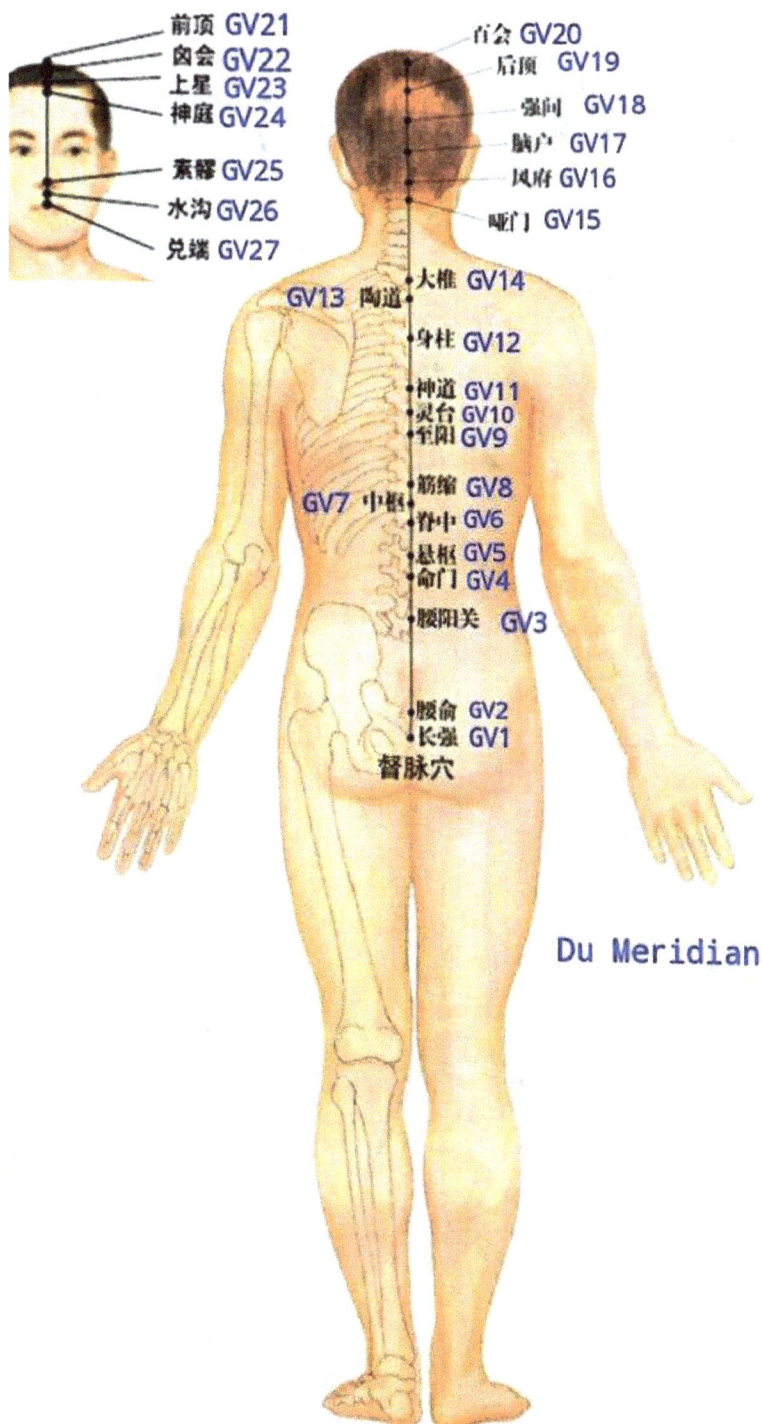

前顶 GV21
囟会 GV22
上星 GV23
神庭 GV24
素髎 GV25
水沟 GV26
兑端 GV27

百会 GV20
后顶 GV19
强间 GV18
脑户 GV17
风府 GV16
哑门 GV15

大椎 GV14
GV13 陶道
身柱 GV12
神道 GV11
灵台 GV10
至阳 GV9
筋缩 GV8
GV7 中枢
脊中 GV6
悬枢 GV5
命门 GV4
腰阳关 GV3
腰俞 GV2
长强 GV1
督脉穴

Du Meridian

25

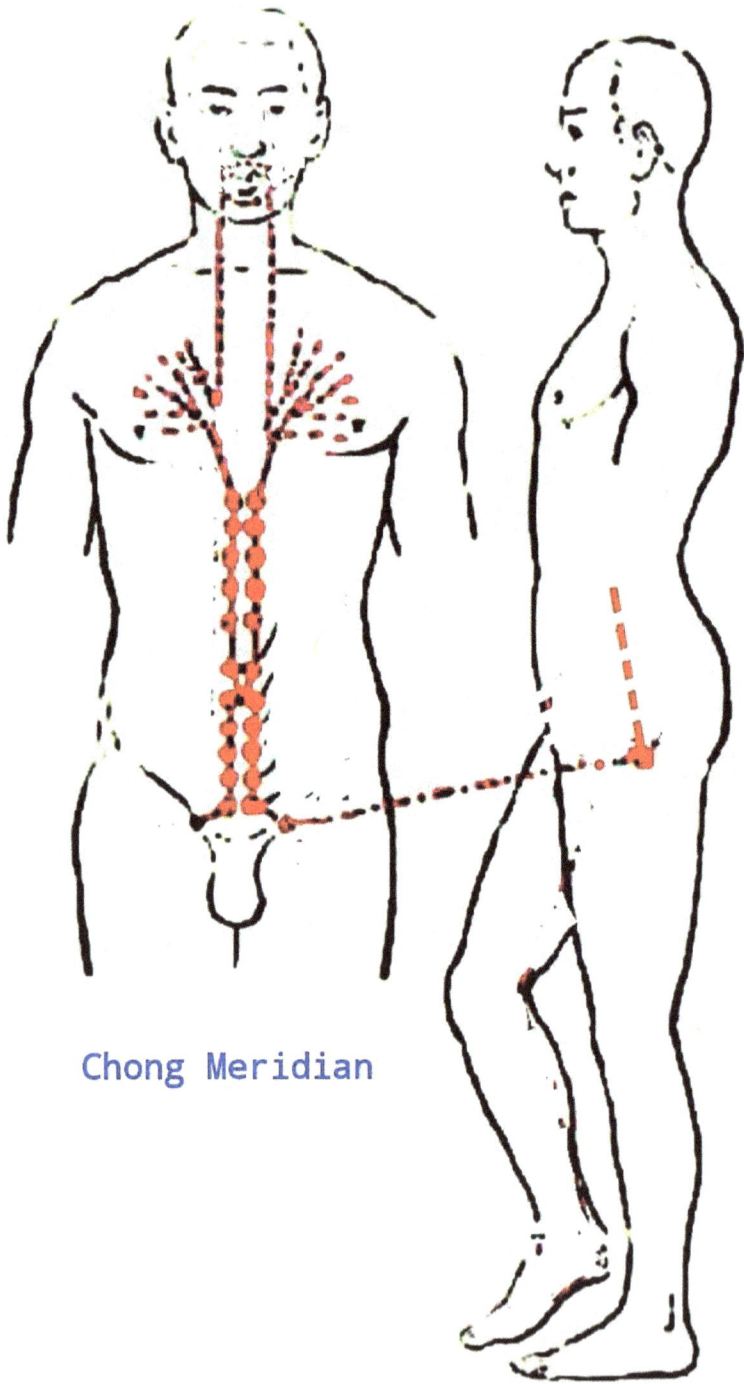

Chong Meridian

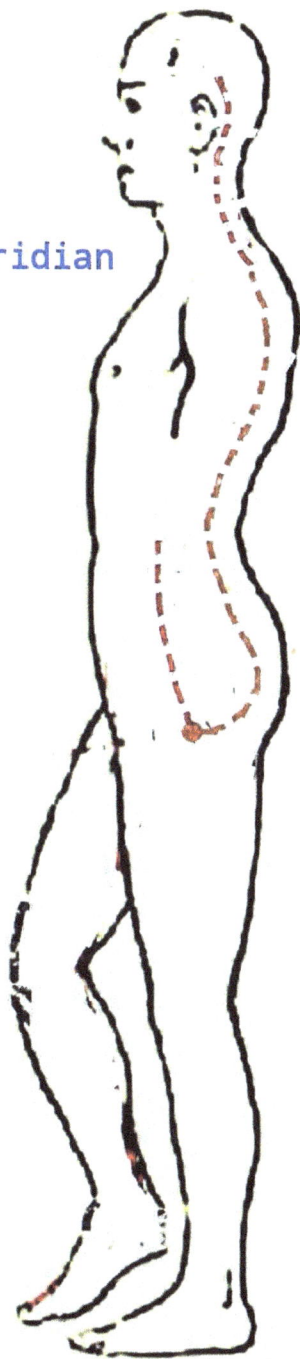

Ji Meridian

References

1. Xiaoguang L. Opening up a new field of modern medical research 2. J Altern Complement Integr Med. 2020; 6:121. Available: https://www.heraldopenaccess.us/openaccess/opening-up-a-new-field-of-modern-medical-research-2

2. Xiaoguang L. Opening up a New Field of Modern Medical Research 3. Global Journal of Medical Research (K) Volume XXI Issue I Version I, Year 2021. Available: https://medicalresearchjournal.org/index.php/GJMR/article/view/2362

3. Li Xiaoguang, The Previously Unknown Secrets of the Human Body, American Academic Press, 2021.

Paper 2: Opening up a New Field of Modern Medical Research 2

This paper was published in the Journal of Alternative, Complementary & Integrative Medicine in October 2020. DOI: 10.24966/ACIM-7562/100121. Citation: Xiaoguang L (2020) Opening up a New Field of Modern Medical Research 2. J Altern Complement Integr Med 6:121

Abstract

Modern medicine tells us that the human body is an organism composed of heart, lung, liver, kidney, spleen, stomach, brain, nerves, muscles, bones, blood vessels, blood and so on, while Traditional Chinese Medicine believes that besides these tissues and organs, the human body still has another part of the structure, Traditional Chinese Medicine calls them Jing Luo and Shu Xue. Jing Luo means the longitudinal line of the human body and the accompanying net, translated into English Meridians and Collaterals. Shu Xue means holes distributed on Jing Luo and outside Jing Luo, because stimulating Shu Xue's position by acupuncture, massage and other methods can cure diseases, so Shu Xue is translated into English acupuncture point, abbreviated as acupoint or point. Meridians and acupoints are the special knowledge of the human body structure in Traditional Chinese Medicine. Traditional Chinese Medicine not only draws the distribution map of the meridians and acupoints in the human body, but also has been using them to treat diseases for thousands of years. There are hundreds of these acupoints, stimulating each one by acupuncture, massage or other methods will have a special effect on the human body and can treat various diseases. But what effect does stimulating every acupoint have on the human body so that it can treat various diseases? The discussion of Traditional Chinese Medicine is vague and incomprehensible, and can not be proved by experiments.

According to the author's research for more than 30 years, this paper makes a clear and accurate exposition of the effects on the human body and diseases that can be treated with acupoint massage. These statements can be proved by experiments, so they are believed to be reliable. It is hoped that meridians, acupoints and massage therapy can be incorporated into modern medicine and become a part of modern medicine after being proved by others through experiments.

Massaging acupoints can not only treat many diseases that are difficult to cure with drugs, but also have simple methods and low cost.

Keywords

Physiology, traditional Chinese medicine, meridian, acupoint, massage, blood, ligament

Introduction

Medicine is not only a science to study the structure and laws of the human body, but also a technology to treat and prevent diseases. In ancient times, different regions used to have different medicine, they had different understanding of the human body and adopted different treatment methods for diseases. However, in modern times, European medicine has achieved rapid development with the help of modern scientific and technological progress, and has soon been accepted by all countries in the world to become world medicine and gradually developed into modern medicine. At present, the research and understanding of the human body in modern medicine has been very thorough and meticulous, reaching the molecular level. Since modern medicine has such a thorough and detailed understanding of the human body, in theory, most diseases of the human body should be cured, but the actual situation is not the case. There are still a large number of diseases that modern medicine is powerless and difficult to cure, even a considerable number of which are seemingly uncomplicated diseases. So what is the reason? The reason is that the current modern medicine has defects and deficiencies in understanding the laws of human body. Meridians and acupoints are very important parts. According to thousands of years' experience of Traditional Chinese Medicine and the author's research, a large number of diseases in the human body are related to meridians and acupoints, which can be treated through meridians and acupoints. Unfortunately, modern medicine knows nothing about this. It is hoped that more people can devote themselves to the research of meridians and acupoints. This will be a promising field.

There are many meridians and acupoints of the human body described in traditional Chinese medicine, this paper discusses the effects on the human body and diseases that can be treated of massaging some acupoints on Du Meridian, Chong Meridian, Ren Meridian and bladder Meridian

The meridian drawn in the following picture is the so-called Du Meridian in Traditional Chinese Medicine.

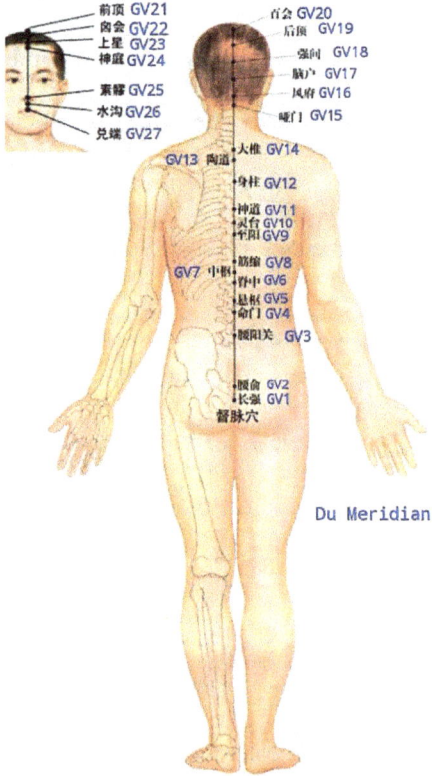

Du Meridian

The meridian drawn in the following picture is the so-called Chong meridian in Traditional Chinese Medicine.

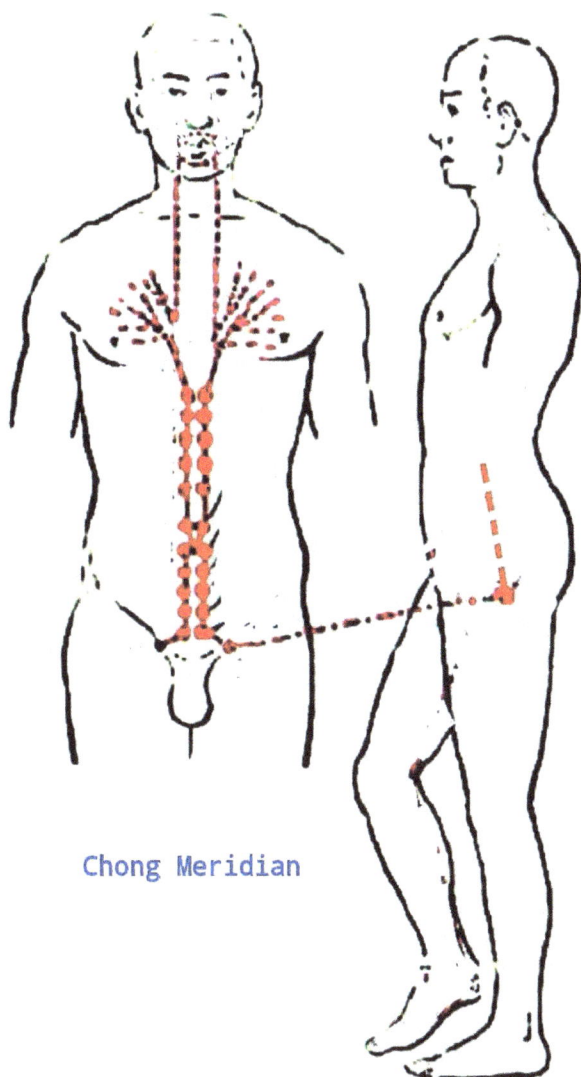

Chong Meridian

The meridian drawn in the following picture is the so-called Ren Meridian and

Bladder Meridian of Foot-Taiyang in Traditional Chinese Medicine.

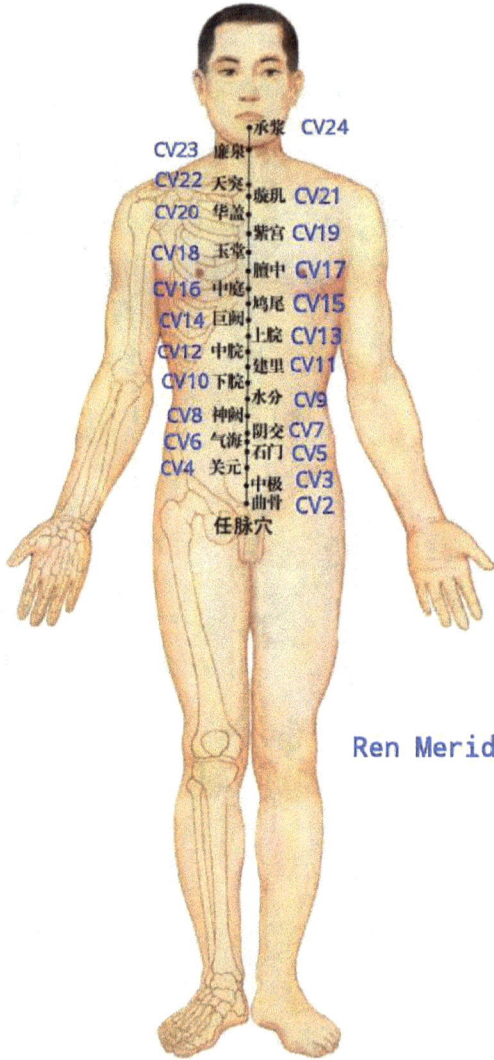

承浆 CV24
CV23 廉泉
CV22 天突 璇玑 CV21
CV20 华盖 紫宫 CV19
CV18 玉堂 膻中 CV17
CV16 中庭 鸠尾 CV15
CV14 巨阙 上脘 CV13
CV12 中脘 建里 CV11
CV10 下脘 水分 CV9
CV8 神阙 阴交 CV7
CV6 气海 石门 CV5
CV4 关元 中极 CV3
曲骨 CV2
任脉穴

Ren Meridian

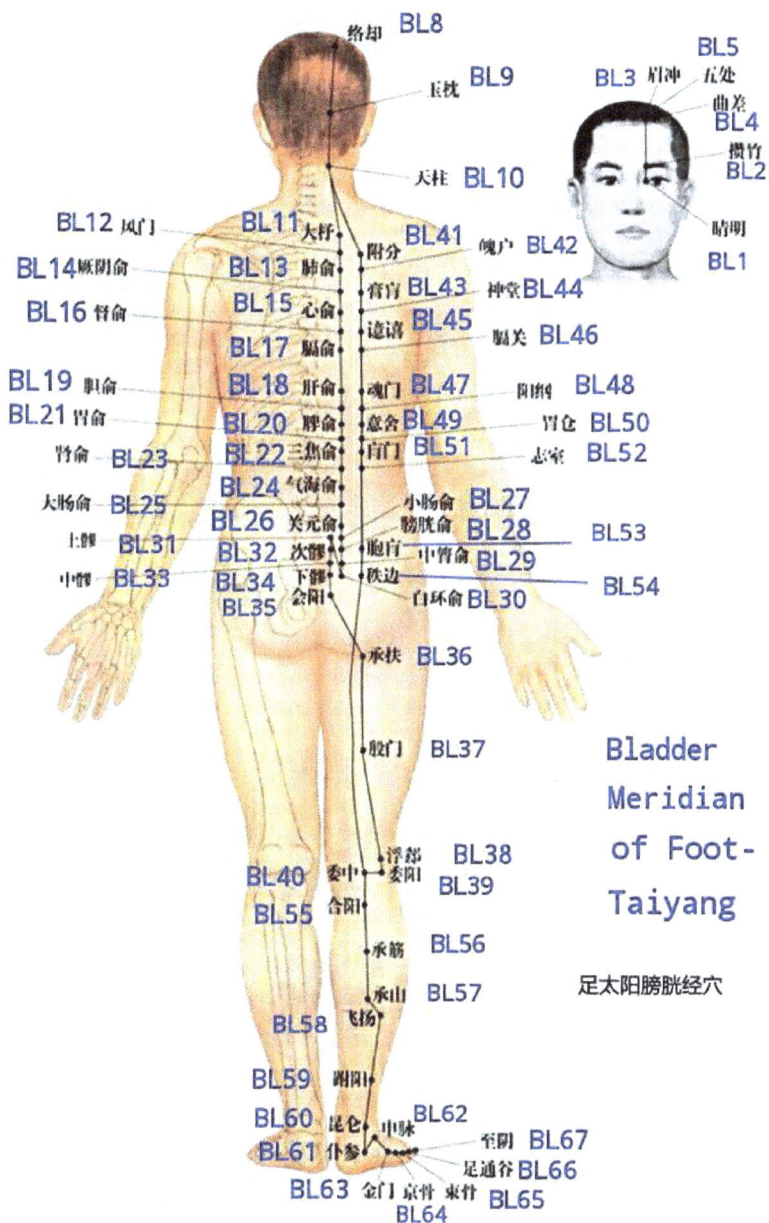

BL8 络却
BL9 玉枕
BL3 眉冲 BL5 五处
曲差 BL4
攒竹 BL2
睛明 BL1

BL10 天柱
BL11 大杼
BL12 风门
BL14 厥阴俞
BL13 肺俞
BL16 肾俞
BL15 心俞
BL17 膈俞
BL19 胆俞
BL18 肝俞
BL21 胃俞
BL20 脾俞
BL23 肾俞
BL22 三焦俞
BL25 大肠俞
BL24 气海俞
BL31 上髎
BL26 关元俞
BL33 中髎
BL32 次髎
BL34 下髎
BL35 会阳
BL41 附分
BL42 魄户
BL43 膏肓
BL44 神堂
BL45 譩譆
BL46 膈关
BL47 魂门
BL48 阳纲
BL49 意舍
BL50 胃仓
BL51 肓门
BL52 志室
BL27 小肠俞
BL28 膀胱俞
BL29 中膂俞
BL30 白环俞
BL53 胞肓
BL54 秩边

BL36 承扶
BL37 殷门

BL38 浮郄
BL39 委阳
BL40 委中
BL55 合阳
BL56 承筋
BL57 承山
BL58 飞扬
BL59 跗阳
BL60 昆仑
BL61 仆参
BL62 申脉
BL63 金门
BL64 京骨
BL65 束骨
BL66 足通谷
BL67 至阴

Bladder Meridian of Foot-Taiyang

足太阳膀胱经穴

Stimulating the acupoints with acupuncture, massage, electricity, cold, heat and other methods will have effects on the human body. The author used massage in his research. The method of massaging acupoints can be either pressing the acupoints with fingers or other things, or rubbing the acupoints with fingers. The interesting thing is that even if you press your finger on the acupoint, no pressure, no friction, will also have the same effect, even through thin clothes can be. Dozens of times or tens of seconds can be used every time. The ones who are physically strong and have certainty about the nature of the disease and the choice of acupoints can be more, while those who are young, old, weak or uncertain about the nature of the disease and the choice of acupoints can be less. It starts to work after the massage, the effect will continue for 7 hours and 40 minutes, and then stop. If you fall asleep in the middle, the period of sleep will not be included in the 7 hours and 40 minutes, because the effect will stop temporarily after you fall asleep and resume after you wake up. For example, when you massage acupoints at 7 o'clock in the evening and fall asleep at 10 o'clock, the effect will stop. When you wake up at 6 o'clock in the morning, the effect will resume again, and then continue until 10:40. The effect of stimulating acupoints is not always manifested very well every time due to various factors, for example, for some reason, stimulating acupoints with opposite effects at the same time can offset the effect, because there are many acupoints in the human body that are stimulated to produce opposite effects.

There are about ten acupoints above Mingmen acupoint GV4 on Du Meridian, which are associated with heart, lung, spleen, stomach, liver, kidney, large intestine, small intestine, gallbladder and bladder respectively, and control the blood flowing into heart, lung, spleen, stomach, liver, kidney, large intestine, small intestine, gallbladder and bladder respectively. A healthy body requires that the blood flowing into the above-mentioned organs is appropriate, so that the function of each organ can be normal, otherwise too little blood flows into the above-mentioned organs, it will lead to the decline of the function of the above-mentioned organs, the reduction of heat production and chills, which is what Traditional Chinese Medicine calls Yang deficiency, such as heart Yang deficiency, lung Yang deficiency and so on. On the contrary, if too much blood flows into the above-mentioned organs, it will lead to hyper-function of these organs, fever, inflammation, pain, diarrhea, bleeding, and so on. Different organs will have different manifestations. Which is what Traditional Chinese Medicine calls Yang excess, for example, heart Yang excess, Lung Yang excess and so on. Massage, pat and stimulation of these acupoints will increase the blood flowing into the corresponding organs, which can respectively treat the diseases caused by insufficient blood supply to various organs, that is, Yang deficiency. But it is not suitable for the opposite situation, that is, Yang excess, which should be banned. As for how to reduce the blood flowing into various organs and treat diseases caused by excessive blood flowing into various organs, that is, Yang excess, please see the Paper 3 "Opening up a New Field of Modern Medical Research 1" in this book or the author's book "The Previously Unknown Secrets of the Human

Body" published by American Academic Press. However which acupoint corresponds to which internal organ, it still needs to be studied in more detail.

There are about ten acupoints on the section of Chong meridian which is located on the surface of chest and abdomen, which are connected with heart, lung, spleen, stomach, liver, kidney, large intestine, small intestine, gallbladder and bladder respectively, and control the blood flowing from heart, lung, spleen, stomach, liver, kidney, large intestine, small intestine, gallbladder and bladder to veins respectively. A healthy body requires that the blood flowing from the above-mentioned organs to veins is appropriate, so the functions of the above-mentioned organs can be normal. Otherwise, if too much blood flows from the above-mentioned organs to veins, it will lead to insufficient blood, decreased function, decreased heat production and chills in each organ, which is called Yin excess in Traditional Chinese Medicine. On the other hand, if there is too little blood flowing out of the above-mentioned organs, it will cause the blood circulation of the above-mentioned organs to be blocked and the above-mentioned organs to be congested, which is what Traditional Chinese Medicine calls Yin deficiency. Massaging, beating and stimulating these acupoints can increase the blood flowing out from the above-mentioned organs, and can treat diseases caused by too little blood flowing out from the above-mentioned organs, that is, Yin deficiency. But it is not suitable for the opposite situation and should be prohibited. As for how to reduce the blood flowing into veins from the above-mentioned organs and treat diseases caused by excessive blood flowing out from the above-mentioned organs, that is, Yin excess, please see Paper 3 "Opening up a New Field of Modern Medical Research 1" in this book and the author's book "The Previously Unknown Secrets of the Human Body" published by American Academic Press. However which acupoint corresponds to which internal organ, it still needs to be studied in more detail.

The acupoints on the branch of the Bladder Meridian of Foot-Taiyang located on the waist and back near the Du Meridian, such as BL13, BL15, BL18, BL23, etc. and the acupoints on the section of Ren Meridian located on the chest and abdomen (except shenque acupoint CV8) are associated with heart, lung, spleen, stomach, liver, kidney, large intestine, small intestine, gallbladder and bladder respectively, and respectively control the tension of ligaments used to fix the positions of various visceral organs. A healthy body requires that the tension of the ligaments of each visceral organ is appropriate, so the body will be normal. On the other hand, if the tension of the ligaments of each visceral organ is too large or too small, people will feel uncomfortable, and the body will be abnormal, while insufficient tension of the ligaments is the cause of the sagging of the visceral organs. Stimulating these acupoints by massaging or beating will increase the tension of the ligaments of each visceral organ. As for how to reduce the tension of ligaments in each internal organs, please see Paper 3 "Opening up a New Field of Modern Medical Research 1" and the author's book "The Previously Unknown Secrets of the Human Body" published by American Academic Press.

References

1. Liu Yanchi, Basic Theory of Traditional Chinese Medicine, Jiangxi Science and Technology Press, China, 1987.

2. Lun Xin, Yi Wei, The Theory of Meridians and Acupoints, Science and Technology Literature Publishing House, China, 2006.

3. Li, Xiaoguang. 2020. Opening up a New Field of Modern Medical Research 1.

4. Li Xiaoguang, The Previously Unknown Secrets of the Human Body, American Academic Press, 2021.

Paper 3: Opening up a New Field of Modern Medical Research 1

This paper was published in the Preprints of osf website in September, 2020. For some reason, it is now invisible.

Abstract

Modern medicine tells us that the human body is an organism composed of heart, lung, liver, kidney, spleen, stomach, brain, nerves, muscles, bones, blood vessels, blood and so on, while traditional Chinese medicine believes that besides these tissues and organs, the human body still has another part of the structure, traditional Chinese medicine calls them Jing Luo and Shu Xue. Jing Luo means the longitudinal line of the human body and the accompanying net, translated into English Meridians and Collaterals. Shu Xue means holes distributed on Jing Luo and outside Jing Luo, because stimulating Shu Xue's position by acupuncture, massage and other methods can cure diseases, so Shu Xue is translated into English acupuncture point, abbreviated as acupoint or point. Meridians and acupoints are the special knowledge of human body structure in traditional Chinese medicine. Traditional Chinese medicine not only draws the distribution map of the meridians and acupoints in the human body, but also has been using them to treat diseases for thousands of years. There are hundreds of these acupoints, stimulating each one by acupuncture, massage or other methods will have a special effect on the human body and can treat various diseases. But what effect does stimulating every acupoint have on the human body so that it can treat various diseases? The discussion of traditional Chinese medicine is vague and incomprehensible, and can not be proved by experiments.

According to the author's research for more than 30 years, this paper makes a clear and accurate exposition of the effects on the human body and diseases that can be treated with acupoint massage. These statements can be proved by experiments, so they are believed to be reliable. It is hoped that meridians, acupoints and massage therapy can be incorporated into modern medicine and become a part of modern medicine after being proved by others through experiments.

Massaging acupoints can not only treat many diseases that are difficult to cure with drugs, but also have simple methods and low cost.

Keywords

Physiology, meridian, acupoint, massage, blood, ligament

Introduction

Medicine is not only a science to study the structure and laws of the human body, but also a technology to treat and prevent diseases. In ancient times, different regions used to have different medicine, they had different understanding of the human body and adopted different treatment methods for diseases. However, in modern times, European medicine has achieved rapid development with the help of modern scientific and technological progress, and has soon been accepted by all countries in the world to become world medicine and gradually developed into modern medicine. At present, the research and understanding of the human body in modern medicine has been very thorough and meticulous, reaching the molecular level. Since modern medicine has such a thorough and detailed understanding of the human body, in theory, most diseases of the human body should be cured, but the actual situation is not the case. There are still a large number of diseases that modern medicine is powerless and difficult to cure, even a considerable number of which are seemingly uncomplicated diseases. So what is the reason? The reason is that the current modern medicine has defects and deficiencies in understanding the laws of human body. Meridians and acupoints are very important parts. According to thousands of years' experience of traditional Chinese medicine and the author's research, a large number of diseases in the human body are related to meridians and acupoints, which can be treated through meridians and acupoints. Unfortunately, modern medicine knows nothing about this. It is hoped that more people can devote themselves to the research of meridians and acupoints. This will be a promising field.

.

The distribution of meridians and acupoints in the human body

Traditional Chinese medicine tells us that the meridians system of the human body is composed of the twelve regular meridians, the eight extraordinary meridians and so on, some of which are distributed in the human body as follows. The figure shows only the part on the body surface, and another part enters the body and is connected with internal organs.

Lung Meridian of Hand-Taiyin   (Lung Meridian for short)

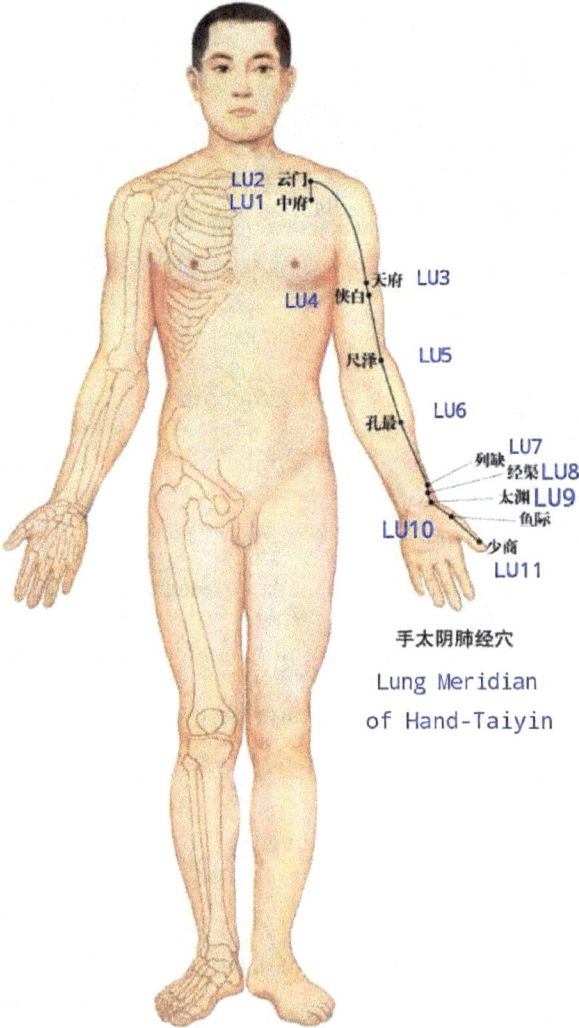

LU2 云门
LU1 中府
天府 LU3
LU4 侠白
尺泽 LU5
孔最 LU6
列缺 LU7
经渠 LU8
太渊 LU9
鱼际
LU10
少商 LU11

手太阴肺经穴
Lung Meridian
of Hand-Taiyin

Figure 1   Lung Meridian is connected with lung and large intestine.

Large Intestine Meridian of Hand-Yangming　(Large Intestine Meridian for short)

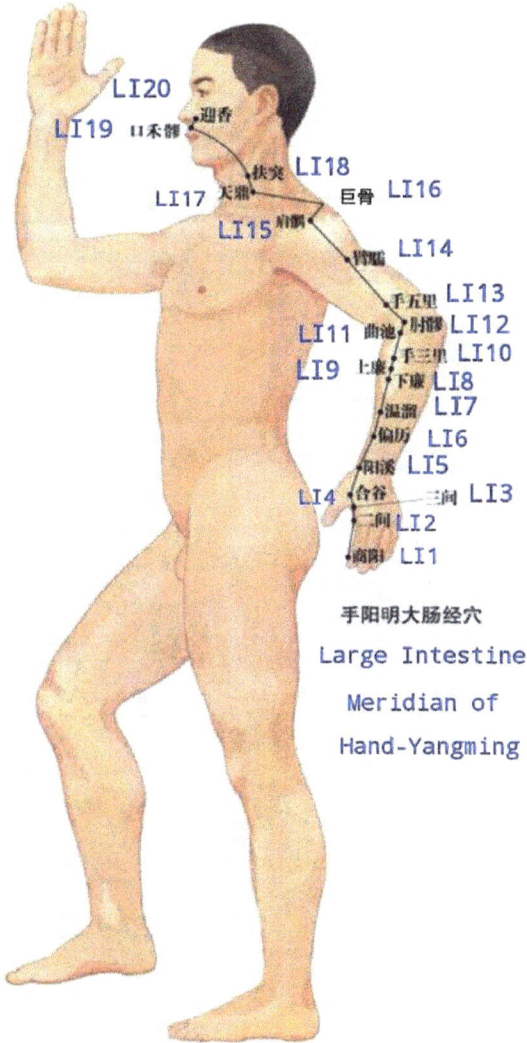

Figure 2　Large Intestine Meridian is connected with large intestine and lung.

Heart Meridian of Hand-Shaoyin   (Heart Meridian for short)

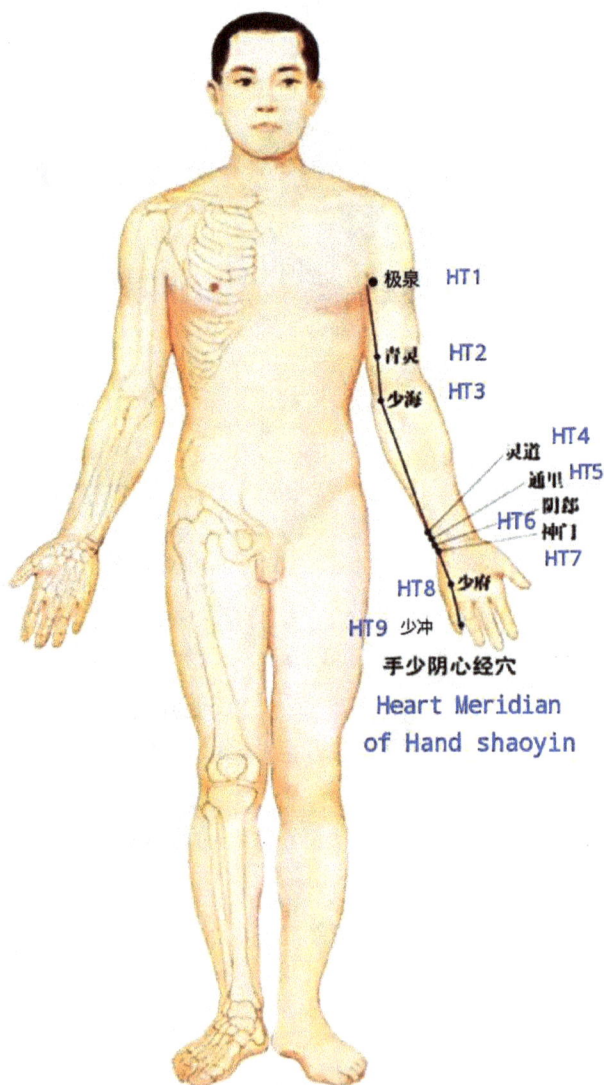

极泉 HT1
青灵 HT2
少海 HT3
灵道 HT4
通里 HT5
阴郄 HT6
神门 HT7
少府 HT8
HT9 少冲

手少阴心经穴
Heart Meridian
of Hand shaoyin

Figure 3   Heart Meridian is connected with heart and small intestine.

Small Intestine Meridian of Hand-Taiyang (Small Intestine Meridian for short)

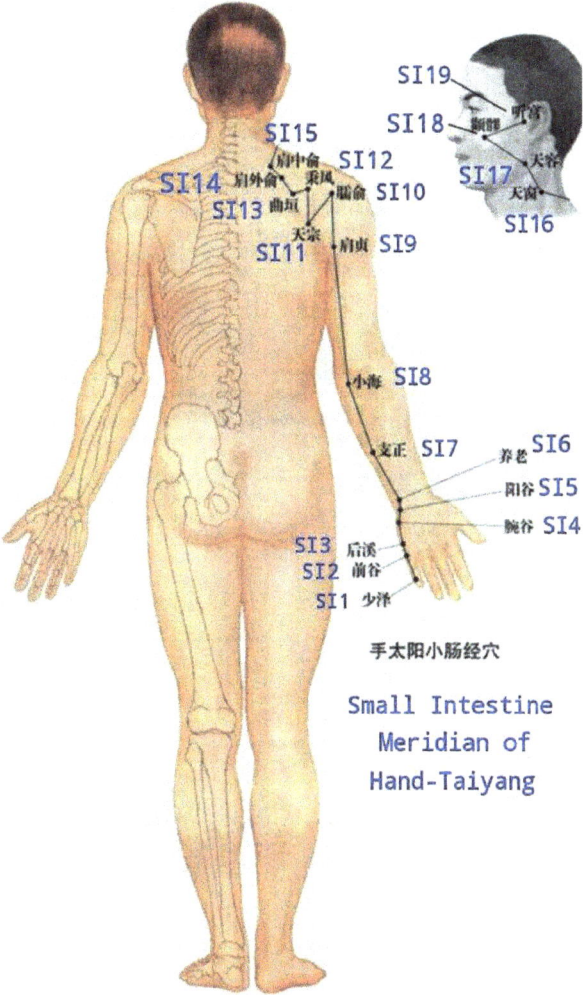

Figure 4 Small Intestine Meridian is connected with small intestine and heart.

Spleen Meridian of Foot-Taiyin   (Spleen Meridian for short)

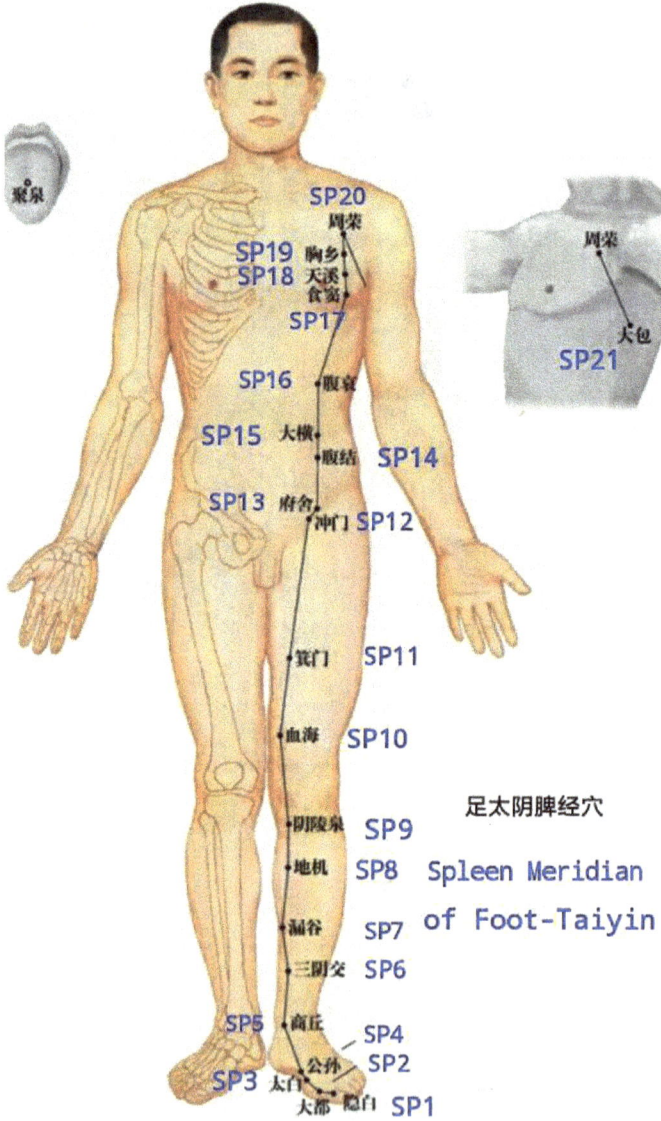

Figure 5   Spleen Meridian is connected with spleen and stomach.

Stomach Meridian of Foot-Yangming   (Stomach Meridian for short)

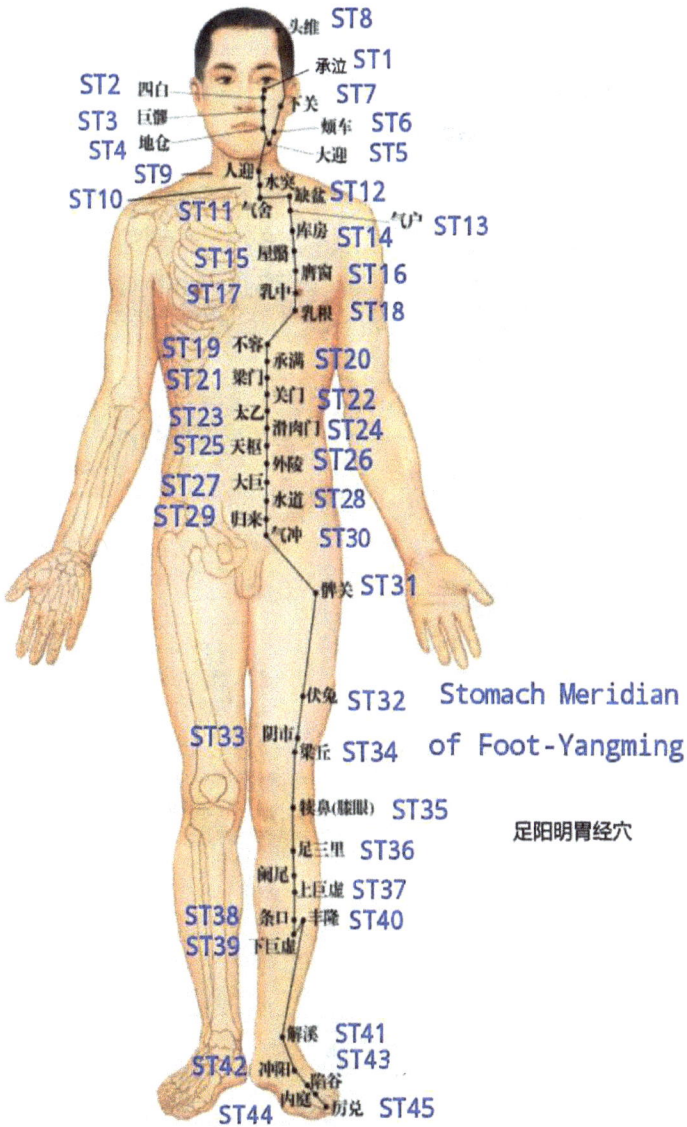

Figure 6   Stomach Meridian is connected with stomach and spleen.

Liver Meridian of Foot-Jueyin (Liver Meridian for short)

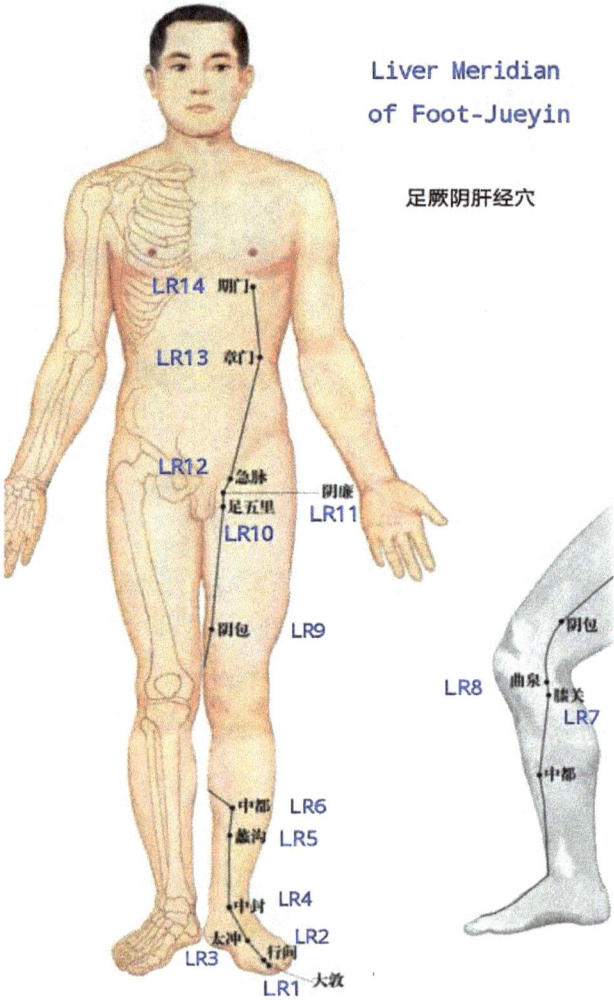

Liver Meridian of Foot-Jueyin

足厥阴肝经穴

LR14 期门
LR13 章门
LR12 急脉
阴廉 LR11
足五里
LR10
阴包 LR9
LR8 曲泉 膝关 LR7
中都 LR6
蠡沟 LR5
中封 LR4
太冲 LR2
LR3 行间
LR1 大敦
阴包
曲泉 膝关 LR7
中都

Figure 7 Liver Meridian is connected with liver and gallbladder.

Gallbladder Meridian of Foot- Shaoyang   (Gallbladder Meridian for short)

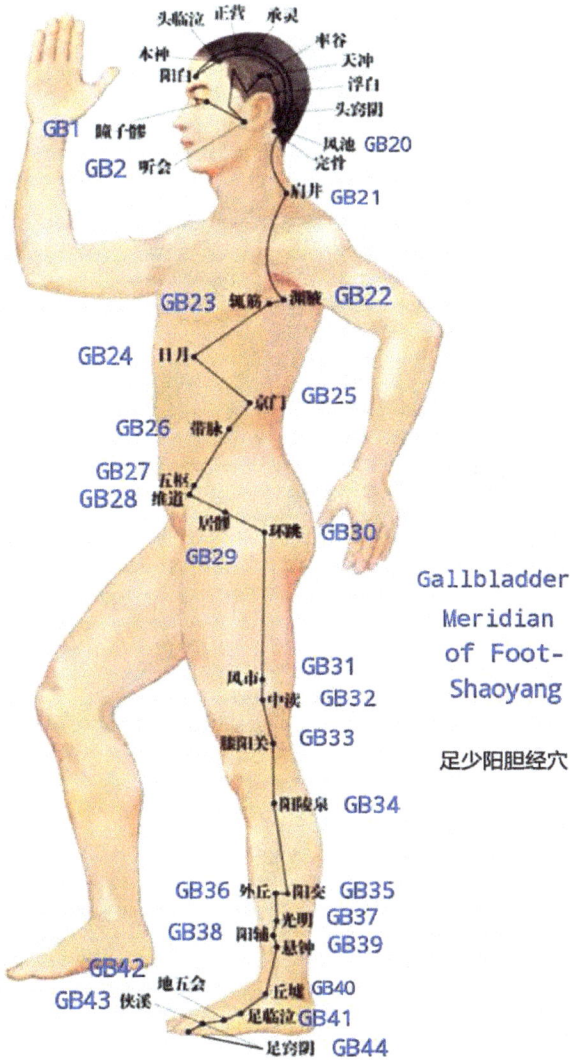

Figure 8   Gallbladder Meridian is connected with gallbladder and liver.

Kidney Meridian of Foot-Shaoyin (Kidney Meridian for short)

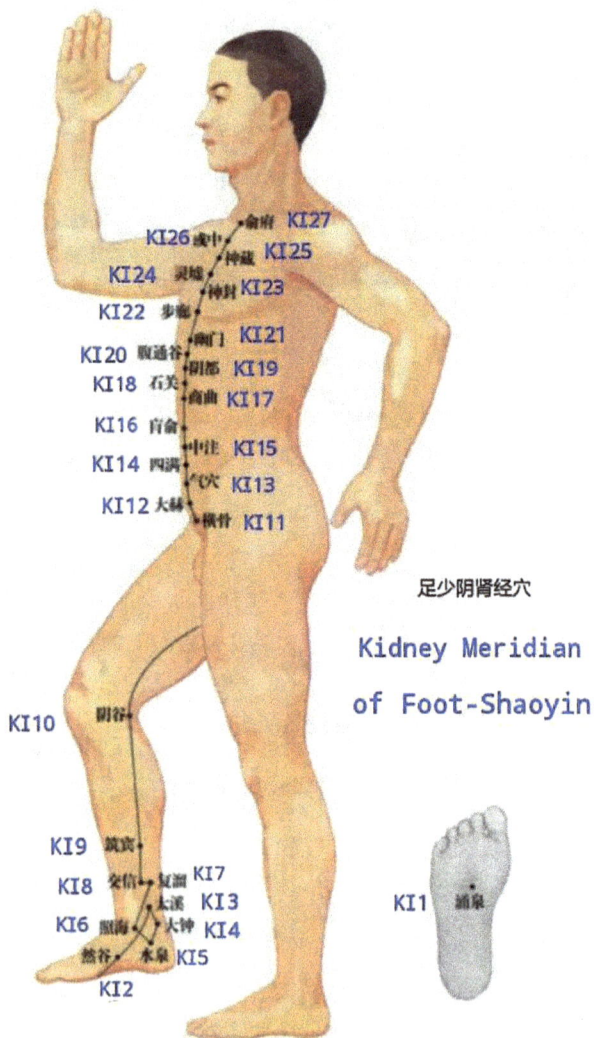

Figure 9 Kidney Meridian is connected with kidney and bladder.

Bladder Meridian of Foot-Taiyang　(Bladder Meridian for short)

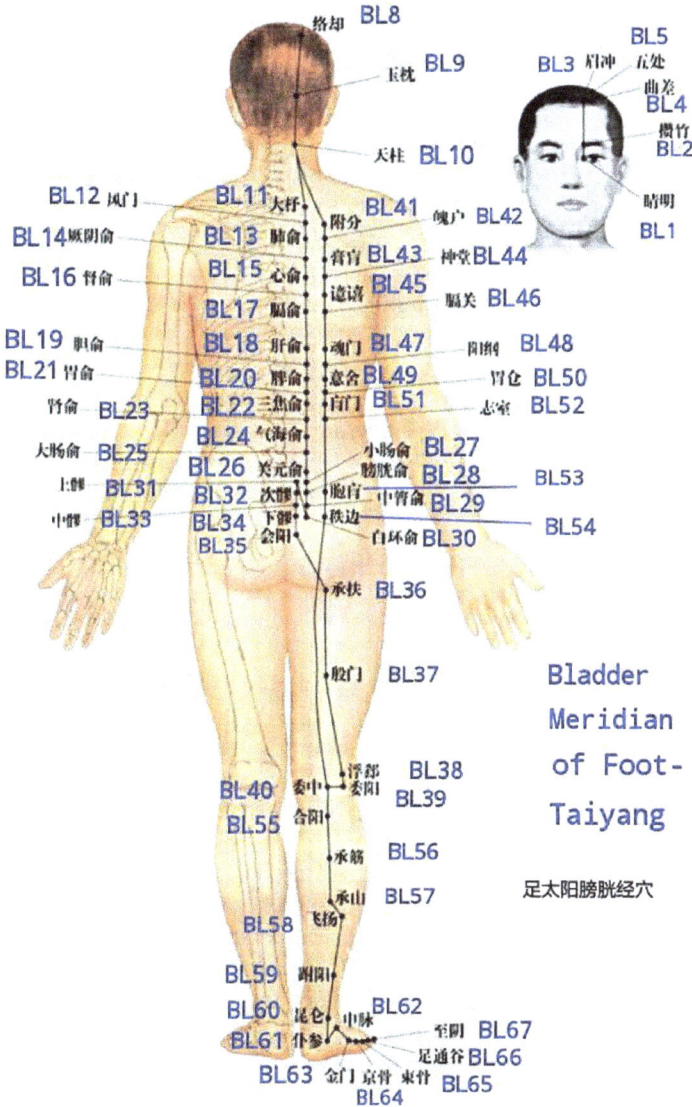

Figure 10　Bladder Meridian is connected with bladder and kidney.

The effect on the human body and diseases that can be treated of massaging some acupoints on the above meridians.

Stimulating acupoints with acupuncture, massage, electricity, cold, heat and other methods will have effects on the human body. The author used massage in his research. The method of massaging acupoints can be either pressing the acupoints with fingers or other things, or rubbing the acupoints with fingers. The interesting thing is that even if you press your finger on the acupoint, no pressure, no friction, will also have the same effect, even through thin clothes can be. Dozens of times or tens of seconds can be used every time. The ones who are physically strong and have certainty about the nature of the disease and the choice of acupoints can be more, while those who are young, old, weak or uncertain about the nature of the disease and the choice of acupoints should be less. It starts to work after the massage, the effect will continue for 7 hours and 40 minutes, and then stop. If you fall asleep in the middle, the period of sleep will not be included in the 7 hours and 40 minutes, because the effect will stop temporarily after you fall asleep and resume after you wake up. For example, when you massage acupoints at 7 o'clock in the evening and fall asleep at 10 o'clock, the effect will stop. When you wake up at 6 o'clock in the morning, the effect will resume again, and then continue until 10:40. The effect of stimulating acupoints is not always manifested very well every time due to various factors, for example, for some reason, stimulating acupoints with opposite effects at the same time can offset the effect, because there are many acupoints in the human body that are stimulated to produce opposite effects.

1. Massaging the acupoints LU4 or LU3 on Lung Meridian of Hand-Taiyin (Figure 1) can simultaneously reduce blood flowing from pulmonary artery to lung and from lung to pulmonary vein, and increase the tension of ligaments in the lung, it can be used for treating diseases caused by excessive blood flowing from pulmonary artery to lung and from lung to pulmonary vein and insufficient tension of ligaments in the lung, but it is inappropriate for the opposite situation and should be prohibited.

2. Massaging the acupoints LU6 or LU2 on Lung Meridian of Hand-Taiyin (Figure 1) will simultaneously increase the blood flowing from the pulmonary artery into the lung and from the lung into the pulmonary vein and reduce the tension of ligaments in the lung, it can treat diseases caused by insufficient blood flowing from the pulmonary artery into the lung and from the lung into the pulmonary vein and excessive tension of ligaments in the lung, but it is inappropriate for the opposite situation and should be prohibited.

3. Massaging the acupoints LI8, LI9 or LI13 on Large Intestine Meridian of Hand-Yangming (Figure 2 and Figure 11) will simultaneously reduce the blood flowing from the artery into the large intestine and from the large intestine into the vein, and increase the tension of ligaments in the large intestine, it can treat diseases caused by excessive blood flowing from the artery into the large intestine and from the large intestine into the vein and insufficient tension of ligaments in the large intestine, but it is inappropriate for the opposite situation and should be

prohibited.

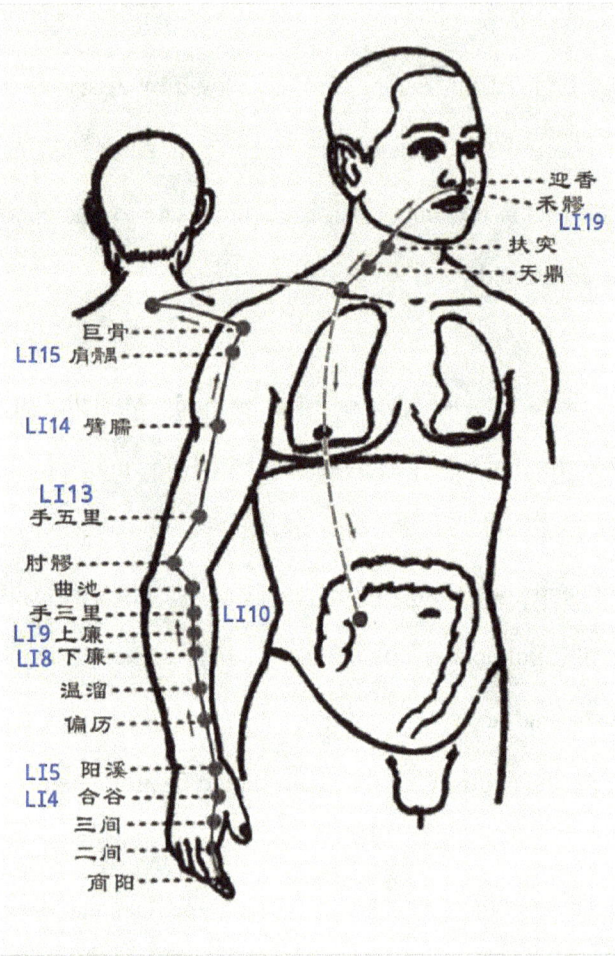

Figure 11

4. Massaging the acupoints LI5, LI10, LI14, LI15 or LI19 on Large Intestine Meridian of Hand-Yangming (Figure 11, Figure 12 and Figure 13) can

simultaneously increase the blood flowing from the artery to the large intestine and from the large intestine to the vein and reduce the tension of ligaments in the large intestine, it can treat diseases caused by insufficient blood flowing from the artery to the large intestine and from the large intestine to the vein and excessive tension of ligaments in the large intestine, but it is inappropriate for the opposite situation and should be prohibited.

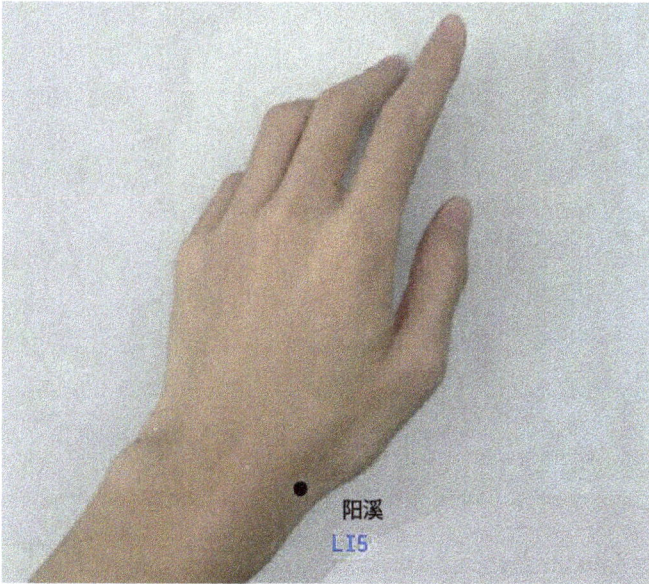

Figure 12

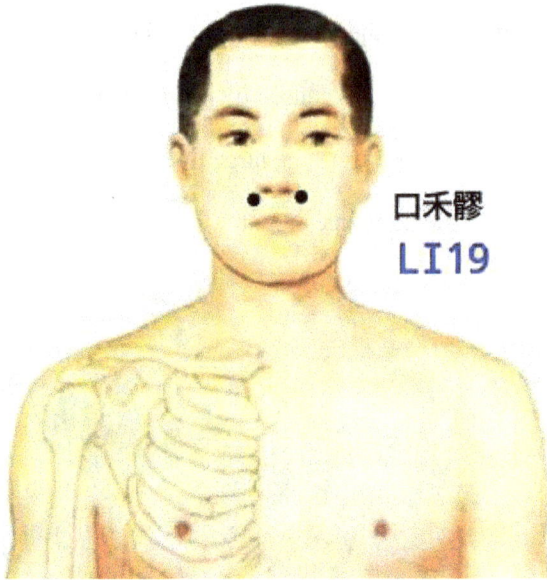

口禾髎
LI19

Figure 13

5. Massaging the acupoints HT8 or HT2 on Heart Meridian of Hand-Shaoyin (Figure 3 and Figure 14) will simultaneously increase the blood flowing from the coronary artery into the myocardium and from the myocardium into the vein and reduce the tension of ligaments in the heart, it can treat diseases caused by insufficient blood flowing from the coronary artery into the myocardium and from the myocardium into the vein and excessive tension of ligaments in the heart, but it is inappropriate for the opposite situation and should be prohibited.

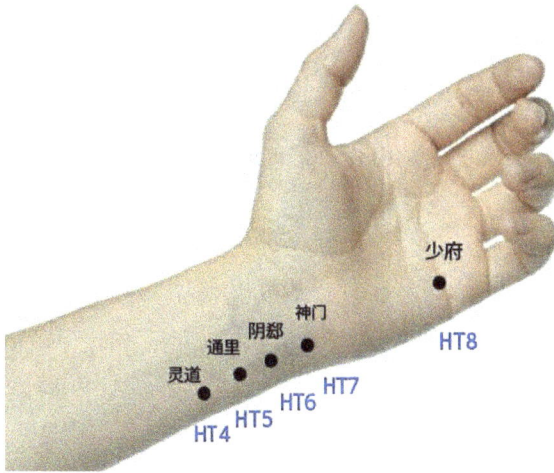

Figure 14

6. Massaging the acupoints HT7 or HT4 on Heart Meridian of Hand-Shaoyin (Figure 3 and Figure 14) can simultaneously reduce the blood flowing from the coronary artery into the myocardium and from the myocardium into the vein and increase the tension of ligaments in the heart, it can be used for treating diseases caused by excessive blood flowing from the coronary artery into the myocardium and from the myocardium into the vein and insufficient tension of ligaments in the heart, but it is inappropriate for the opposite situation and should be prohibited.

7. Massaging the acupoints SI2, SI9, SI18 or SI19 on Small Intestine Meridian of Hand-Taiyang (Figure 4, Figure 15 and Figure 16) can simultaneously increase the blood flowing from the artery into the small intestine and from the small

intestine into the vein and reduce the tension of ligaments in the small intestine, it can treat diseases caused by insufficient blood flowing from the artery into the small intestine and from the small intestine into the vein and excessive tension of ligaments in the small intestine, but it is inappropriate for the opposite situation and should be prohibited.

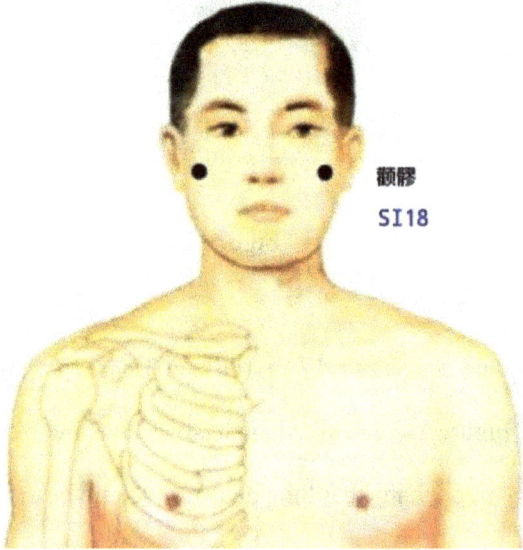

Figure 15

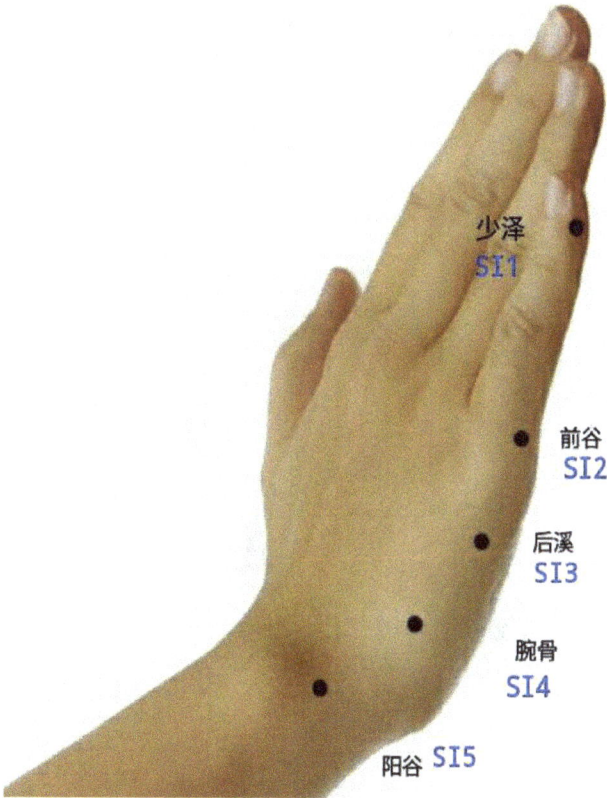

Figure 16

8. Massaging the acupoints SI4, SI6, SI10, SI16 or SI17 on Small Intestine Meridian of Hand-Taiyang (Figure 4, Figure 16 and Figure 17) can simultaneously reduce the blood flowing from the artery into the small intestine and from the small intestine into the vein, increase the tension of ligaments in the small intestine, and can treat diseases caused by excessive blood flowing from the artery into the small intestine and from the small intestine into the vein and

insufficient tension of ligaments in the small intestine, but it is inappropriate for the opposite situation and should be prohibited.

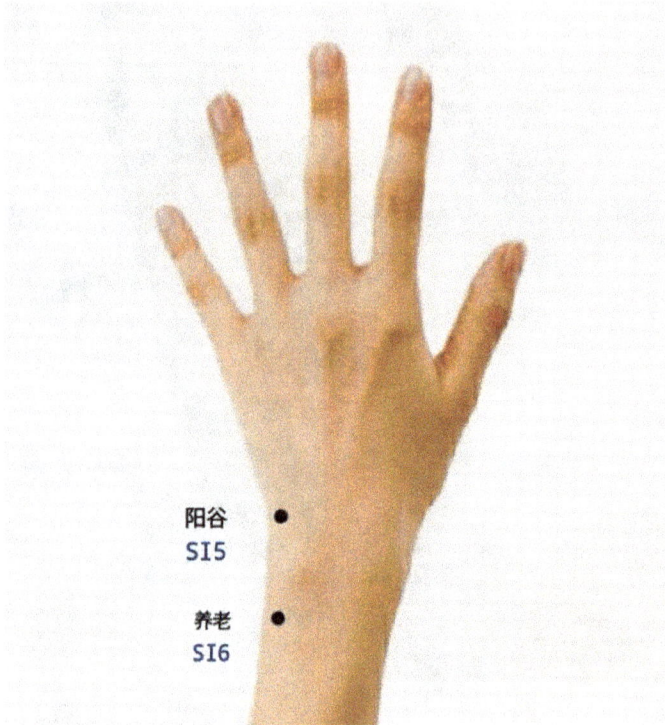

Figure 17

9. Massaging the acupoint SP1 on Spleen Meridian of Foot-Taiyin (Figure 5 and Figure 18) can simultaneously increase blood flowing from the artery to the spleen and from the spleen to the vein and reduce the tension of ligaments in the spleen, it can treat diseases caused by insufficient blood flowing from the artery to the spleen and from the spleen to the vein and excessive tension of ligaments in the spleen, but it is inappropriate for the opposite situation and should be prohibited.

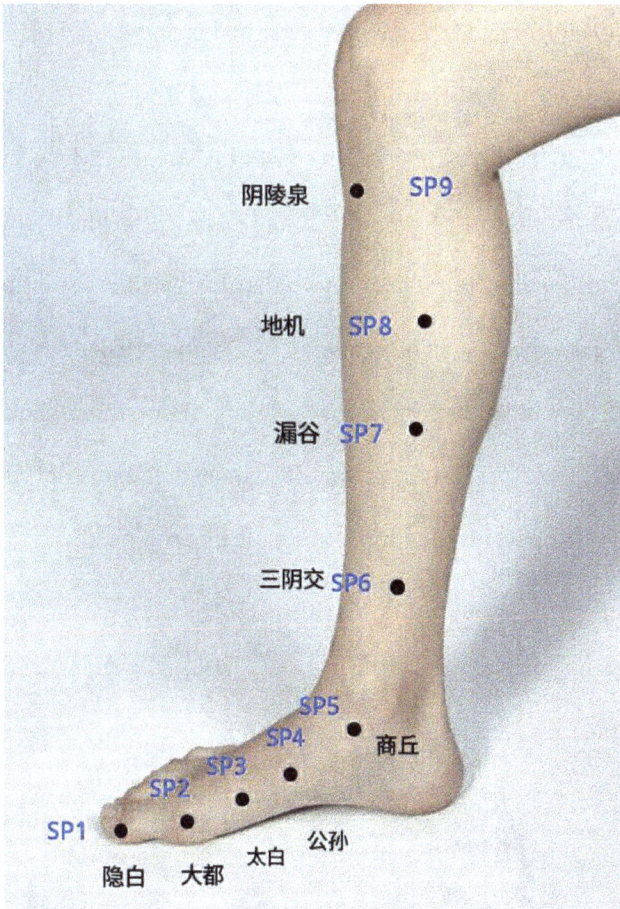

Figure 18

10. Massaging the acupoint SP3 on Spleen Meridian of Foot-Taiyin (Figure 5 and Figure 18) can simultaneously reduce blood flowing from the artery to the spleen and from the spleen to the vein, increase the tension of ligaments in the spleen, and can treat diseases caused by excessive blood flowing from the artery to the spleen and from the spleen to the vein and insufficient tension of ligaments in the

spleen, but it is inappropriate for the opposite situation and should be prohibited.

11. Massaging the acupoints ST7, ST12 or ST44 on Stomach Meridian of Foot-Yangming (Figure 6, Figure 19, Figure 20 and Figure 21) can simultaneously increase the blood flowing from the artery to the stomach and from the stomach to the vein and reduce the tension of ligaments in the stomach, it can treat diseases caused by insufficient blood flowing from the artery to the stomach and from the stomach to the vein and excessive tension of ligaments in the stomach, but it is inappropriate for the opposite situation and should be prohibited.

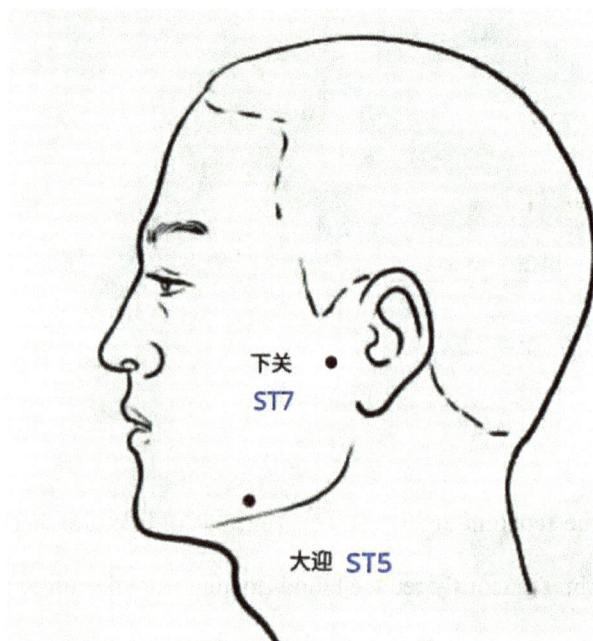

Figure 19

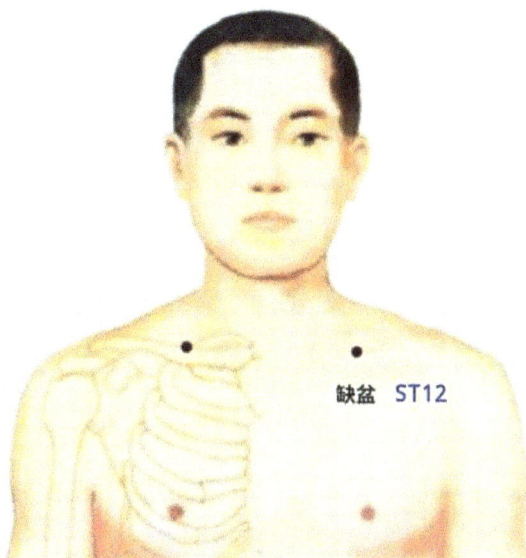

缺盆　ST12

Figure 20

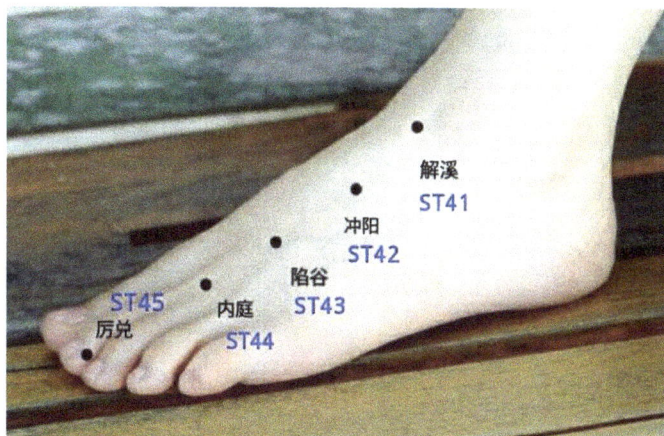

解溪
ST41

冲阳
ST42

陷谷
ST45　　内庭　ST43
厉兑　　　ST44

Figure 21

12. Massaging the acupoint ST42 on Stomach Meridian of Foot-Yangming (Figure 6 and Figure 21) will simultaneously reduce the blood flowing from the artery into the stomach and from the stomach into the vein, increase the tension of ligaments in the stomach, and can treat diseases caused by excessive blood flowing from the artery into the stomach and from the stomach into the vein and insufficient tension of ligaments in the stomach, but it is inappropriate for the opposite situation and should be prohibited.

13. Massaging the acupoint LR1 on Liver Meridian of Foot-Jueyin (Figure 7 and Figure 22) will simultaneously increase the blood flowing from the artery to the liver and from the liver to the vein and reduce the tension of ligaments in the liver, it can treat diseases caused by insufficient blood flowing from the artery to the liver and from the liver to the vein and excessive tension of ligaments in the liver, but it is inappropriate for the opposite situation and should be prohibited.

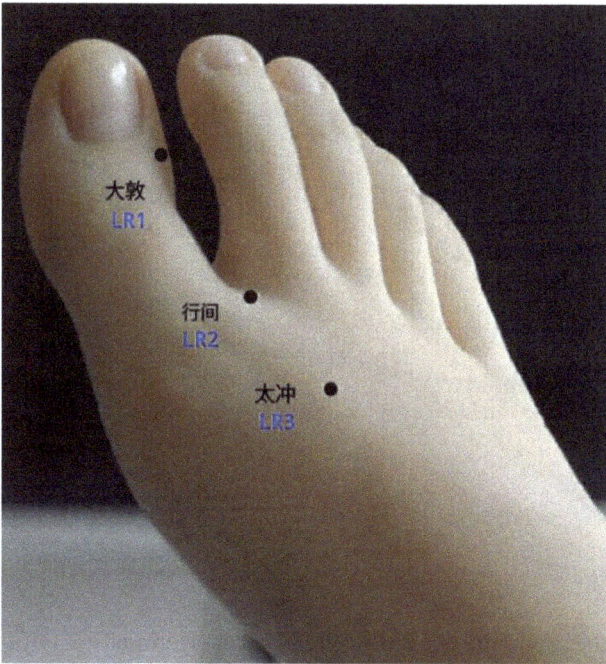

Figure 22

14. Massaging the acupoint LR17 on Liver Meridian of Foot-Jueyin (Figure 7 and Figure 23) will simultaneously reduce the blood flowing from the artery to the liver and from the liver to the vein and increase the tension of ligaments in the liver, it can be used to treat diseases caused by excessive blood flowing from the artery to the liver and from the liver to the vein and insufficient tension of ligaments in the liver, but it is inappropriate for the opposite situation and should be prohibited.

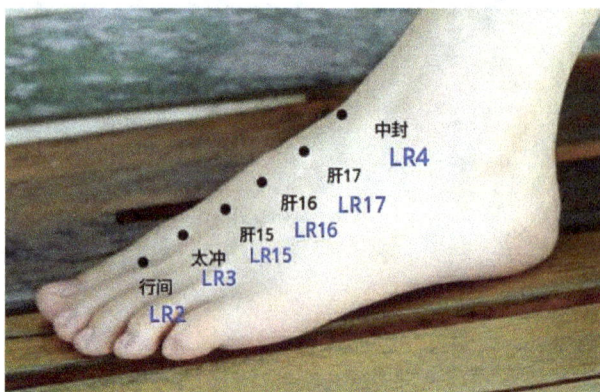

Figure 23

15. Massaging the acupoint GB40 on Gallbladder Meridian of Foot-Shaoyang (Figure 8 and Figure 24) can simultaneously reduce the blood flowing from the artery to the gallbladder and from the gallbladder to the vein and increase the tension of ligaments in the gallbladder, it can be used to treat diseases caused by excessive blood flowing from the artery to the gallbladder and from the gallbladder to the vein and insufficient tension of ligaments in the gallbladder, but it is inappropriate for the opposite situation and should be prohibited.

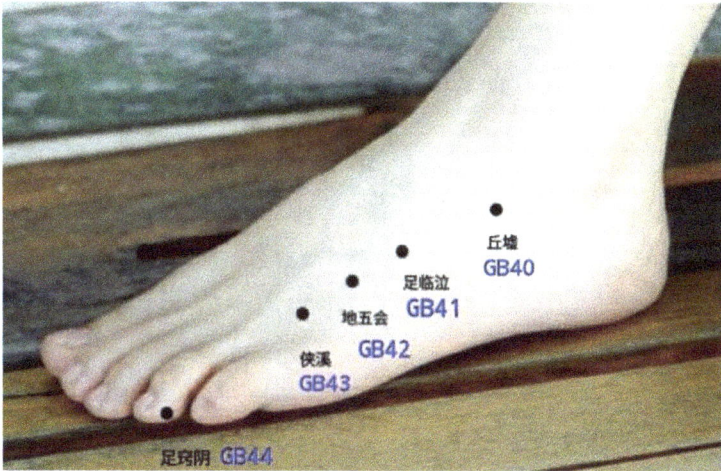

Figure 24

16. Massaging the acupoint GB39 on Gallbladder Meridian of Foot- Shaoyang (Figure 8 and Figure 25) can simultaneously increase blood flowing from the artery to the gallbladder and from the gallbladder to the vein and reduce the tension of ligaments in the gallbladder, it can be used to treat diseases caused by insufficient blood flowing from the artery to the gallbladder and from the gallbladder to the vein and excessive tension of ligaments in the gallbladder, but it is inappropriate for the opposite situation and should be prohibited.

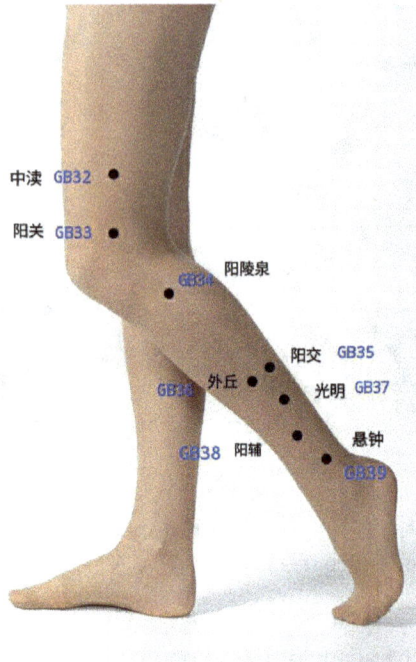

Figure 25

17. Massaging the acupoint KI2 on Kidney Meridian of Foot-Shaoyin (Figure 9 and Figure 26) can simultaneously increase the blood flowing from the artery to the kidney and from the kidney to the vein and reduce the tension of ligaments in the kidney, it can treat diseases caused by insufficient blood flowing from the artery to the kidney and from the kidney to the vein and excessive tension of ligaments in the kidney, but it is inappropriate for the opposite situation and should be prohibited.

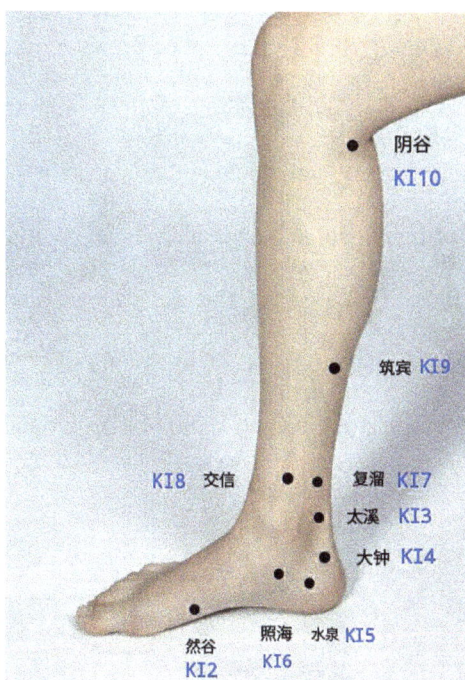

Figure 26

18. Massaging the acupoint KI3 on Kidney Meridian of Foot-Shaoyin (Figure 9 and Figure 26) can simultaneously reduce blood flowing from the artery to the kidney and from the kidney to the vein, increase the tension of ligaments in the kidney, and can treat diseases caused by excessive blood flowing from the artery to the kidney and from the kidney to the vein and insufficient tension of ligaments in the kidney, but it is inappropriate for the opposite situation and should be prohibited.

19. Massaging the acupoints BL1, BL36, BL59 or BL66 on Bladder Meridian of Foot-Taiyang (Figure 10, Figure 27 and Figure 28) can simultaneously increase the blood flowing from the artery to the bladder and from the bladder to the vein and reduce the tension of ligaments in the bladder, it can be used to treat diseases caused by insufficient blood flowing from the artery to the bladder and from the bladder to the vein and excessive tension of ligaments in the bladder, but it is inappropriate for the opposite situation and should be prohibited.

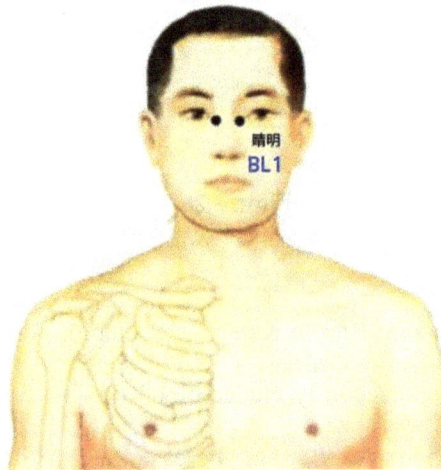

晴明
BL1

Figure 27

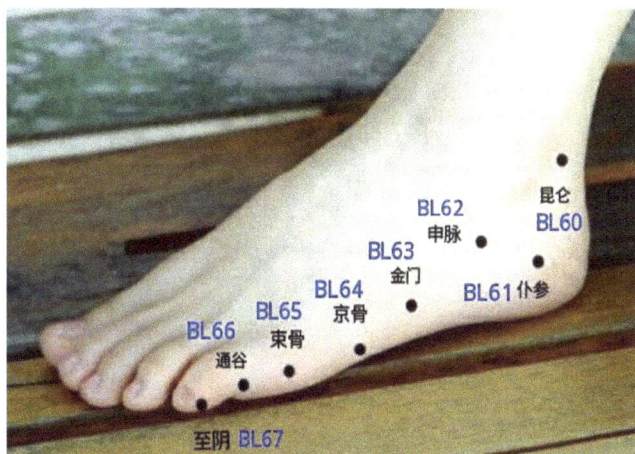

Figure 28

20. Massaging the acupoints BL2, BL10, BL58 or BL64 on Bladder Meridian of Foot-Taiyang (Figure 10, Figure 28 and Figure 29) can simultaneously reduce the blood flowing from the artery into the bladder and from the bladder into the vein, increase the tension of ligaments in the bladder, and can treat diseases caused by excessive blood flowing from the artery into the bladder and from the bladder into the vein and insufficient tension of ligaments in the bladder, but it is inappropriate for the opposite situation and should be prohibited.

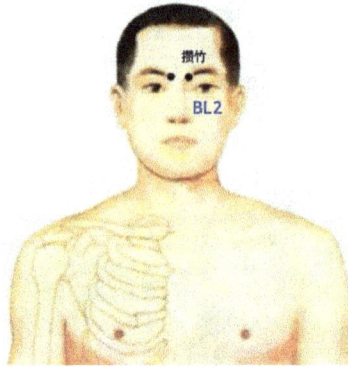

Figure 29

References

1. Liu Yanchi, Basic Theory of Traditional Chinese Medicine, Jiangxi Science and Technology Press, China, 1987.

2. Lun Xin, Yi Wei, The Theory of Meridians and Acupoints, Science and Technology Literature Publishing House, China, 2006.

Paper 4: Opening up a New Field of Modern Medical Research 3

.

This paper was published in Global Journal of Medical Research (K) Interdisciplinary in February 2021. Retrieved from https://medicalresearchjournal.org/index.php/GJMR/article/view/2362. Citation: Xiaoguang, L. (2021). Opening up a New Field of Modern Medical Research 3. Global Journal Of Medical Research (K) Volume XXI Issue I Version I,0 Year 2021.

Abstract

This paper is a continuation of "Opening up a New Field of Modern Medical Research 1" published in Preprints of osf and "Opening up a New Field of Modern Medical Research 2" published in the Journal of Alternative, Complementary & Integrative Medicine.

Modern medicine tells us that the human body is an organism composed of heart, lung, liver, kidneys, spleen, stomach, brain, nerves, muscles, bones, blood vessels, blood, and so on. At the same time, Traditional Chinese Medicine believes that besides these tissues and organs, the human body still has another part of the structure, Traditional Chinese Medicine calls them Jing Luo and Shu Xue. Jing

Luo means the longitudinal line of the human body and the accompanying net, translated into English Meridians and Collaterals. Shu Xue means holes distributed on Jing Luo and outside Jing Luo. Because stimulating Shu Xue's position by acupuncture, massage and other methods can cure diseases, so Shu Xue is translated into an English acupuncture point, abbreviated as acupoint or point. Meridians and acupoints are the special knowledge of human body structure in Traditional Chinese Medicine. Traditional Chinese Medicine not only draws the distribution map of the meridians and acupoints in the human body, but also has been using them to treat diseases for thousands of years. There are hundreds of these acupoints, stimulating each one by acupuncture, massage, or other methods will have a special effect on the human body and can treat various diseases. But what effect does stimulating every acupoint have on the human body so that it can treat various diseases? The discussion of Traditional Chinese Medicine is vague and incomprehensible, and can not be proved by experiments.

According to the author's research for more than 30 years, this paper makes a clear and accurate exposition of the effects on the human body and diseases that can be treated with acupoint massage. These statements can be proved by experiments, so they are believed to be reliable. It is hoped that meridians, acupoints, and massage therapy can be incorporated into modern medicine and become a part of modern medicine after being proved by others through experiments.

Massaging acupoints can not only treat many diseases that are difficult to cure with drugs, but also have simple methods and low cost.

Keywords

Physiology, pathology, Traditional Chinese Medicine, meridian, acupoint, massage, electricity, blood.

I. Introduction

Medicine is not only a science that studies the structure and laws of the human body, but also a technology to treat and prevent diseases. In ancient times, different regions used to have different medicine, they had a different understanding of the human body and adopted different treatment methods for diseases. However, in modern times, European medicine has achieved rapid development with the help of modern scientific and technological progress, and has soon been accepted by all countries in the world to become world medicine and gradually developed into modern medicine. At present, the research and understanding of the human body in modern medicine have been very thorough and meticulous, reaching the molecular level. Since modern medicine has such a thorough and detailed understanding of the human body, in theory, most diseases of the human body should be cured, but the actual situation is not the case.   There are still a large number of diseases that modern medicine is powerless and difficult to cure, even a considerable number of which are seemingly uncomplicated diseases. So what is the reason?   The reason is that the current modern medicine has defects and deficiencies in understanding the laws of the human body.

Meridians and acupoints are very important parts. According to thousands of years' experience in Traditional Chinese Medicine and the author's research, a large number of diseases in the human body are related to meridians and acupoints, which can be treated through meridians and acupoints. Unfortunately, modern medicine knows nothing about this. It is hoped that more people can devote themselves to the research of meridians and acupoints. This will be a promising field.

II. The meridians involved in this paper

Traditional Chinese Medicine tells us that the meridians system of the human body is composed of the twelve regular meridians, the eight extraordinary meridians and so on. The following meridians are involved in this paper. The figures show only the part on the body surface, and another part enters the body and is connected with internal organs.

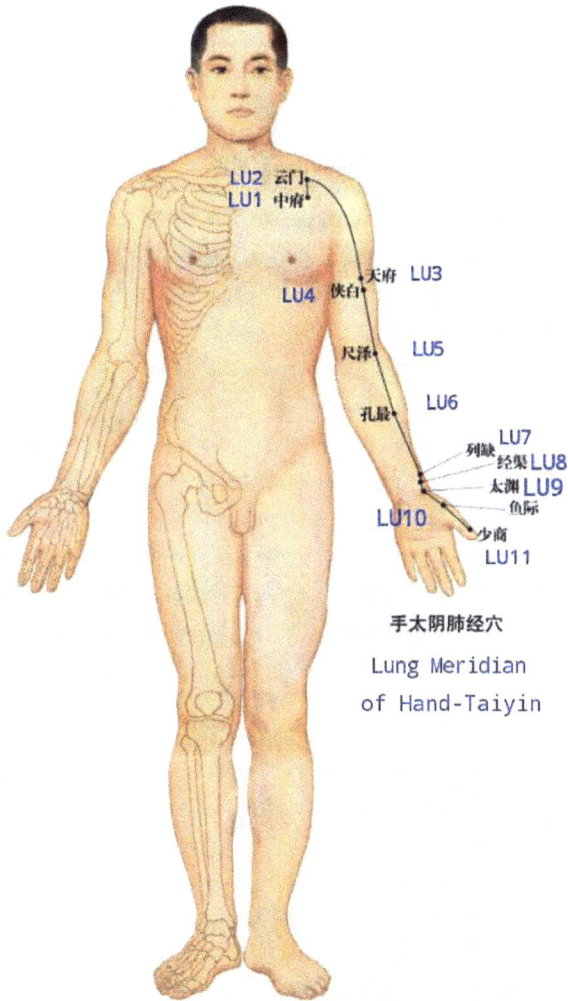

Figure 1 Lung Meridian of Hand-Taiyin (Lung Meridian for short)

Lung Meridian enters the body and connects with the lungs and large intestine.

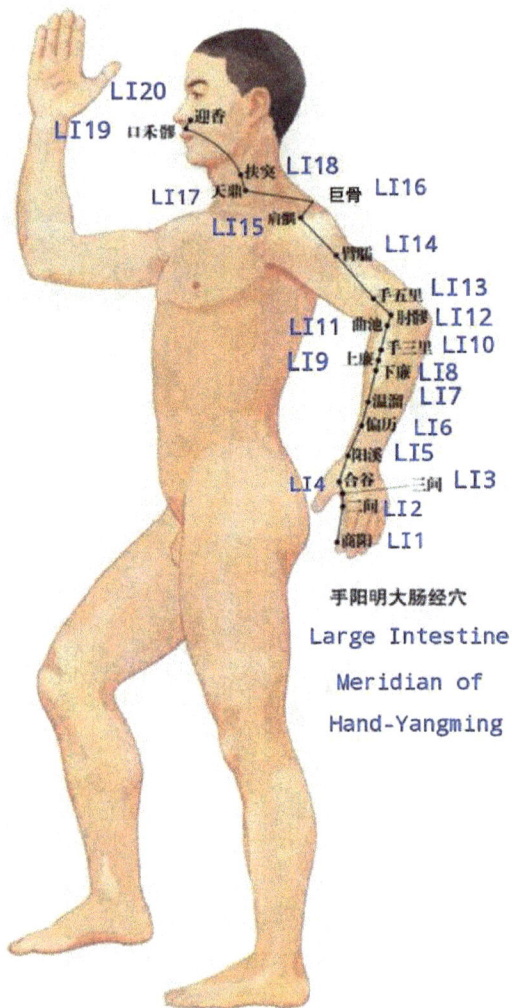

LI20
LI19 口禾髎 迎香
扶突 LI18
LI17 天鼎 巨骨 LI16
LI15 肩髃
臂臑 LI14
手五里 LI13
曲池 肘髎 LI12
LI11 手三里 LI10
LI9 上廉 下廉 LI8
温溜 LI7
偏历 LI6
阳溪 LI5
LI4 合谷 三间 LI3
二间 LI2
商阳 LI1

手阳明大肠经穴
Large Intestine
Meridian of
Hand-Yangming

Figure 2 Large Intestine Meridian of Hand-Yangming (Large Intestine Meridian for short)

Large Intestine Meridian enters the body and connects with the large intestine and lungs.

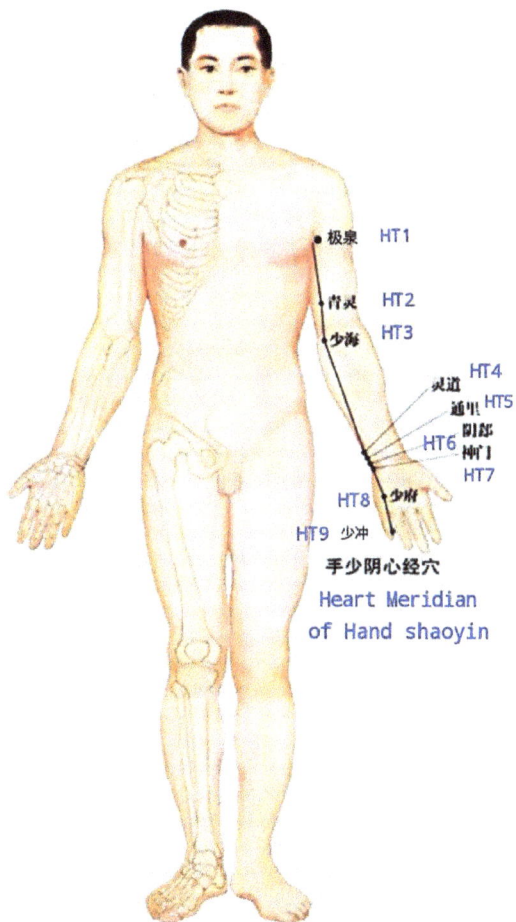

Figure 3　Heart Meridian of Hand-Shaoyin　(Heart Meridian for short)

Heart meridian enters the body and connects with the heart and small intestine.

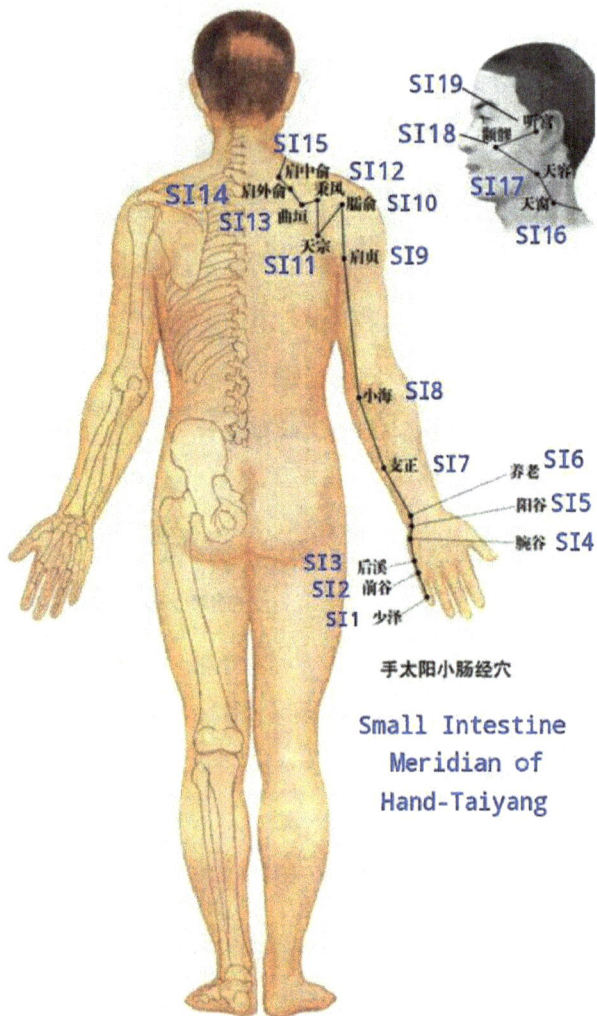

Figure 4 Small Intestine Meridian of Hand-Taiyang (Small Intestine Meridian for short)

Small Intestine Meridian enters the body and connects with the small intestine and heart.

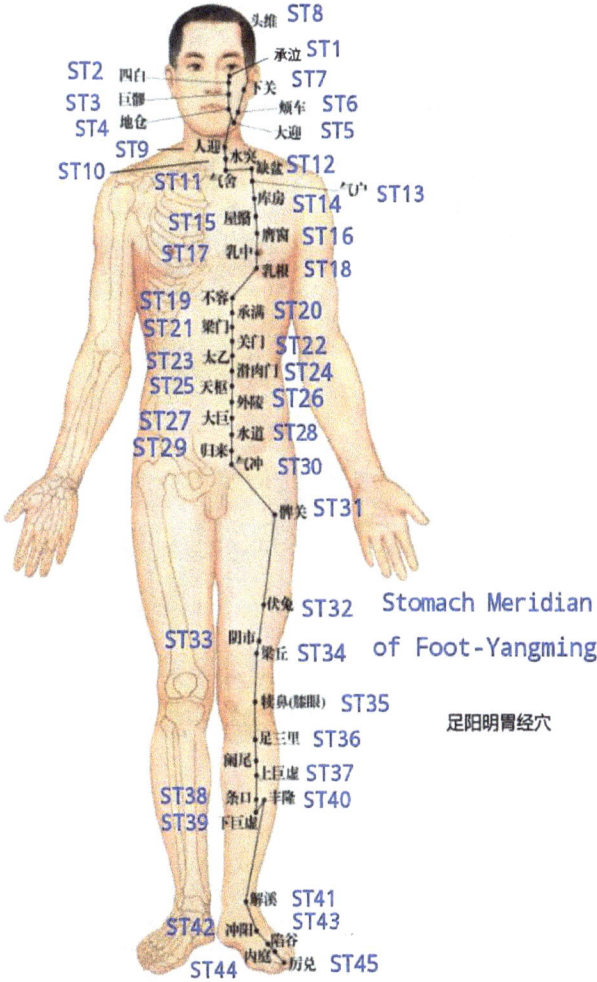

Figure 5   Stomach Meridian of Foot-Yangming   (Stomach Meridian for short)

Stomach Meridian enters the body and connects with the stomach and spleen.

III. The effect on the human body and diseases that can be treated of massaging some acupoints on these five meridians

The following introduces the effects on the human body and the diseases that can be treated by massaging some acupoints on these five meridians. The massage method can be either rubbing on acupoints with fingers, or pressing on acupoints with fingers or other slender or sharp hard objects. Putting your fingers on acupoints without rubbing or pressing can also have effect. Tens of times or seconds at a time. The ones who are physically strong and have certainty about the nature of the disease and the choice of acupoints can be more, while those who are young, old, weak, or uncertain about the nature of the disease and the choice of acupoints should be less. It starts to work after the massaging, the effect will continue for 7 hours and 40 minutes, and then stop. If you fall asleep in the middle, the period of sleep will not be included in the 7 hours and 40 minutes, because the effect will stop temporarily after you fall asleep and resume after you wake up. For example, when you massage acupoints at 7 p.m. and fall asleep at 10 o'clock, the effect will stop. When you wake up at 6 a.m., the effect will resume again, and then continue until 10:40. The effect of massaging acupoints is not always manifested very well every time due to various factors. For example, for some reason, stimulating acupoints with opposite effects at the same time can offset the effect, because there are many acupoints in the human body that are stimulated to produce the opposite effects.

1. Massaging the acupoint LU10 on Lung Meridian of Hand-Taiyin (Figures 1 and 6) can simultaneously increase the blood flowing from pulmonary artery to lungs and from lungs to pulmonary vein, and reduce the electricity of the lungs and large intestine, it can be used to treat diseases caused by insufficient blood flowing from pulmonary artery to lungs and from lungs to pulmonary vein and excessive electricity of the lungs and large intestine, but it is inappropriate for the opposite situation and should be prohibited.

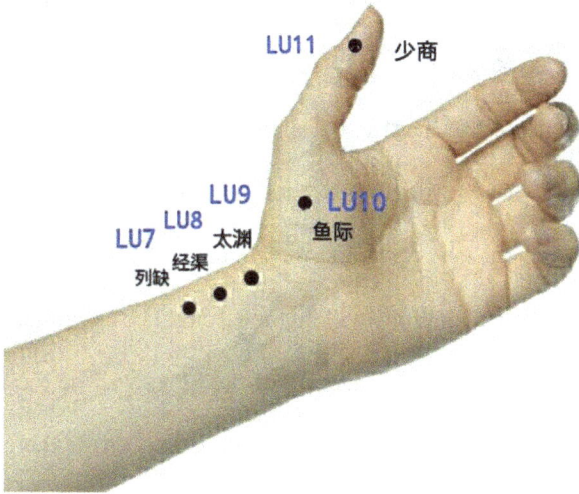

Figure 6   Acupoints on Lung Meridian of Hand-Taiyin

Electricity is called Qi in Traditional Chinese Medicine. Electricity in the lungs is called Lung Qi, electricity in the heart is called Heart Qi, etc. A healthy body not only requires that the blood flowing from the arteries to the internal organs and from the internal organs to the veins be appropriate, not too much or too little, but also requires that the electricity of internal organs be appropriate, not too much or too little, too much or too little will cause abnormal functions of internal organs and make people sick. The diseases caused by too much or too little blood flowing from arteries to internal organs and from internal organs to veins have been mentioned in the previous two papers, this paper will not repeat, but only talks about the diseases caused by too much or too little electricity in internal organs. If the internal organs have too little electricity, their functions will be insufficient and weak. For example, if the electricity of the lungs is insufficient, the function of the lungs will be weak, and people will feel short of breath and breathing weakness. If the electricity of the heart is not enough, the function of the heart will be weak, and people will feel depressed, tired, weak, unresponsive, sleepy, unwilling to speak, and have a low voice. On the contrary, if the internal organs have too much electricity, their functions will be too strong. For example, if there is too much electricity in the lungs, the function of the lungs will be too strong, and people will feel wheezing, chest tightness, cough and so on. If there is too much electricity in the heart, the function of the heart will be too strong, and people will feel suffocated in the chest, excited, palpitation, easily frightened, upset and insomnia. Other organs are similar to this.

2. Massaging the acupoint LU8 on Lung Meridian of Hand-Taiyin (Figures 1 and 6) can simultaneously reduce the blood flowing from pulmonary artery to lungs and from lungs to pulmonary vein, and increase the electricity in the lungs and

large intestine. It can be used to treat diseases caused by excessive blood flowing from pulmonary artery to lungs and from lungs to pulmonary vein and insufficient electricity in the lungs and large intestine, but it is inappropriate for the opposite situation and should be prohibited.

3. Massaging the acupoints LI3 or LI18 on the Large Intestine Meridian of Hand-Yangming (Figures 2 and 7) can simultaneously increase the blood flowing from artery to large intestine and from large intestine to vein and reduce the electricity of the lungs and large intestine, it can treat diseases caused by insufficient blood flowing from artery to large intestine and from large intestine to vein and excessive electricity of the lungs and large intestine. Similarly, it is inappropriate for the opposite situation and should be prohibited.

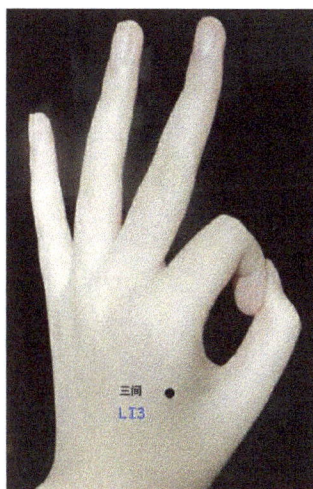

Figure 7   Acupoints on Large Intestine Meridian of Hand-Yangming

4. Massaging the acupoints LI7 or LI17 on the Large Intestine Meridian of Hand-Yangming (Figures 2 and 8) can simultaneously reduce the blood flowing from artery to large intestine and from large intestine to vein, increase the electricity of the lungs and large intestine, and can treat diseases caused by excessive blood flowing from artery to large intestine and from large intestine to vein and insufficient electricity of the lungs and large intestine. Similarly, it is inappropriate for the opposite situation and should be prohibited.

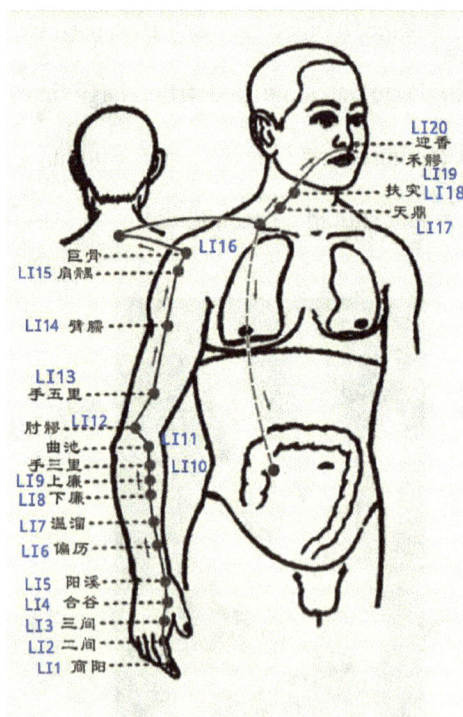

Figure 8   Acupoints on Large Intestine Meridian of Hand-Yangming

5. Massaging the acupoint HT6 on the Heart Meridian of Hand-Shaoyin (Figures 3 and 9) can simultaneously reduce the blood flowing from the coronary artery into the myocardium and from the myocardium into the vein, increase the electricity of the heart and small intestine, and can treat diseases caused by excessive blood flowing from the coronary artery into the myocardium and from the myocardium into the vein and insufficient electricity of the heart and small intestine. Similarly, it is not suitable for the opposite situation and should be prohibited.

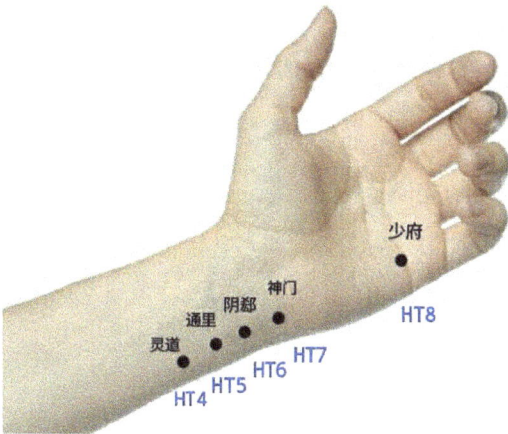

Figure 9   Acupoints on Heart Meridian of Hand-Shaoyin

6. Massaging the acupoint HT5 on the Heart Meridian of Hand-Shaoyin (Figures 3 and 9) can simultaneously increase the blood flowing from the coronary artery into the myocardium and from the myocardium into the vein and reduce the

electricity of the heart and small intestine, it can treat diseases caused by insufficient blood flowing from the coronary artery into the myocardium and from the myocardium into the vein and excessive electricity of the heart and small intestine. Similarly, it is inappropriate for the opposite situation and should be prohibited.

7. Massaging the acupoint SI1 on the Small Intestine Meridian of Hand-Taiyang (Figures 4 and 10) can simultaneously increase the blood flowing from the artery into the small intestine and from the small intestine into the vein and reduce the electricity of the heart and small intestine, it can treat diseases caused by insufficient blood flowing from the artery into the small intestine and from the small intestine into the vein and excessive electricity of the heart and small intestine. Similarly, it is inappropriate for the opposite situation and should be prohibited.

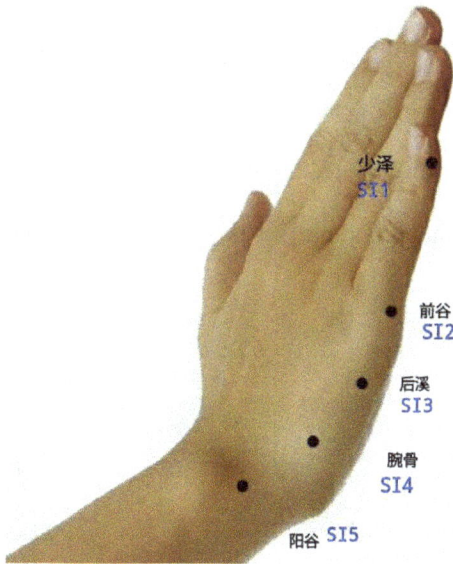

少泽
SI1

前谷
SI2

后溪
SI3

腕骨
SI4

阳谷 SI5

Figure 10　　Acupoints on Small Intestine Meridian of Hand-Taiyang

8. Massaging the acupoint SI5 on the Small Intestine Meridian of Hand-Taiyang (Figures 4 and 10) can simultaneously reduce the blood flowing from the artery into the small intestine and from the small intestine into the vein, increase the electricity of the heart and small intestine, and can treat diseases caused by excessive blood flowing from the artery into the small intestine and from the small intestine into the vein and insufficient electricity of the heart and small intestine. Similarly, it is inappropriate for the opposite situation and should be prohibited.

9. Massaging the acupoints ST43, ST35, ST33, ST10, ST8, ST2, or ST1 on the Stomach Meridian of Foot-Yangming (Figures 5, 11, 12, 13, 14, and 15) can

simultaneously increase the blood flowing from the artery into the stomach and from the stomach into the vein and reduce the electricity of the stomach, it can treat diseases caused by insufficient blood flowing from the artery into the stomach and from the stomach into the vein and excessive electricity of the stomach. Similarly, it is inappropriate for the opposite situation and should be prohibited.

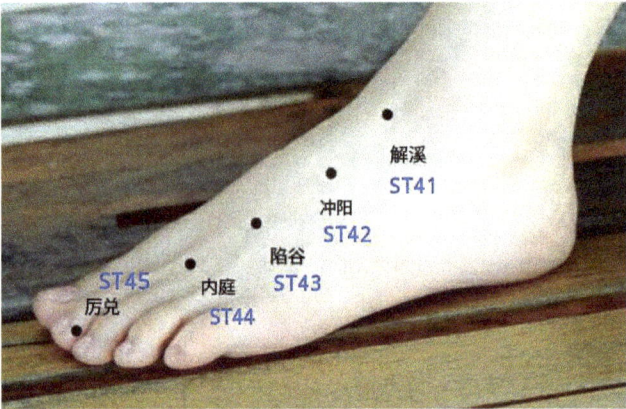

Figure 11　Acupoints on Stomach Meridian of Foot-Yangming

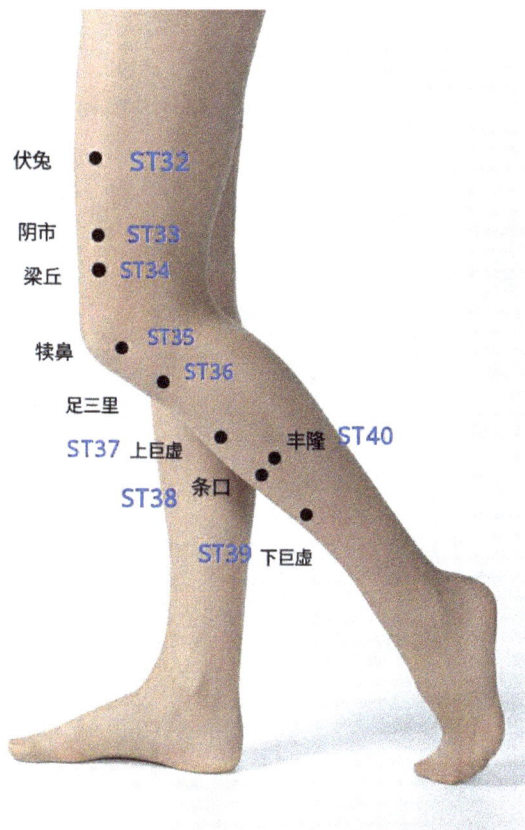

Figure 12   Acupoints on Stomach Meridian of Foot-Yangming

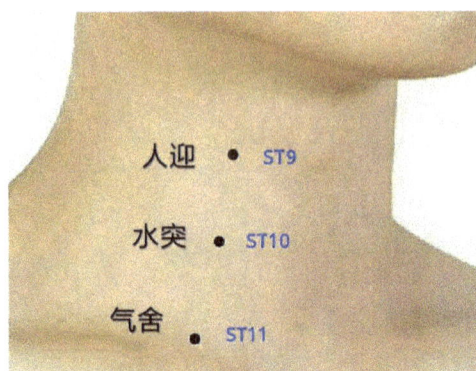

Figure 13　Acupoints on Stomach Meridian of Foot-Yangming

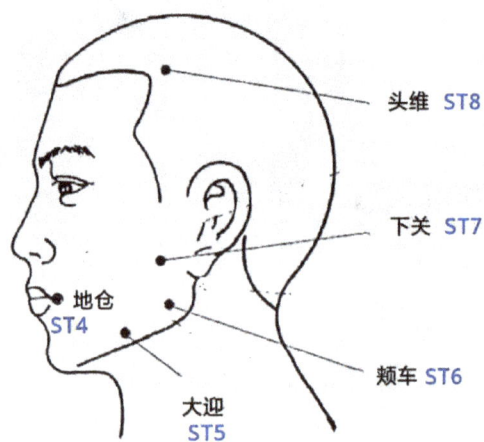

Figure 14　Acupoints on Stomach Meridian of Foot-Yangming

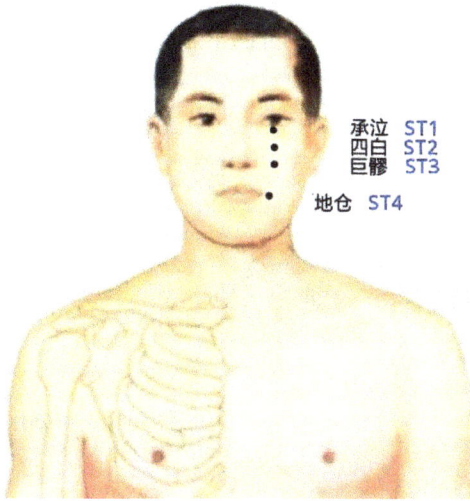

Figure 15   Acupoints on Stomach Meridian of Foot-Yangming

10. Massaging the acupoints ST39, ST34, ST32, ST11, ST5, or ST3 on the Stomach Meridian of Foot-Yangming (Figures 5, 12, 13, 14, and 15) can simultaneously reduce the blood flowing from the artery into the stomach and from the stomach into the vein, increase the electricity of the stomach, and can treat diseases caused by excessive blood flowing from the artery into the stomach and from the stomach into the vein and insufficient electricity of the stomach. Similarly, it is not suitable for the opposite situation and should be prohibited.

Literature

1. Liu Yanchi, Basic Theory of Traditional Chinese Medicine, Jiangxi Science and Technology Press, China, 1987.

2. Lun Xin, Yi Wei, The Theory of Meridians and Acupoints, Science and Technology Literature Publishing House, China, 2006.

3. Li, Xiaoguang. 2020. Opening up a New Field of Modern Medical Research 1.

4. Xiaoguang L (2020) Opening up a New Field of Modern Medical Research 2. J Altern Complement Integr Med 6: 121.

Postscript

The four papers included in this book are only about one-third of the contents of the functions and therapeutic principles of meridians and acupoints discovered by the author, and more contents have been published through another book, The Previously Unknown Secrets of the Human Body. Interested readers can read it.

www.ingramcontent.com/pod-product-compliance
Lightning Source LLC
Chambersburg PA
CBHW050540270326

41926CB00015B/3315